PRAISE FOR JON GORDON AND *EN*

"Since today everybody thinks you're open 24/7, increasing your energy is an important survival strategy. Read Jon Gordon's *Energy Addict* and learn simple, powerful strategies to increase your physical, mental and spiritual energy. Read it so you can go for it!"

—Ken Blanchard, coauthor of *The One Minute Manager* and *Gung Ho!*

"If you often feel like you're out of gas, slowing down, or running on fumes, this book will help you to find the fuel to enliven your life FOR LIFE. Full of great tips, it's an easy, enjoyable, light, and inspiring read. Jon Gordon's mind-body approach to increasing your energy really works!"

—Michael Gerrish, author of *The Mind-Body Makeover Project* and *When Working Out Isn't Working Out*

"*Energy Addict* can help many athletes focus and increase their energy during times of high performance. It's been a great book for all my clients who enjoy the game of golf."

—Cindy Reid, author of *Cindy Reid's Ultimate Guide to Golf for Women* and director of instruction, TPC at Sawgrass, Top-50 Female Instructor 2003

"Read this compelling book and you'll get out of bed, get dressed and wonder why you ever went to bed at all! Rid yourself of Energy Vampires, practice Zoom Focus and, I would add, have a Fierce Conversation. Jon Gordon persuades us that energy acquisition is a skill anyone can learn. Positive energy is contagious. Give yourself and others this powerful infusion."

—Susan Scott, author of *Fierce Conversations, Achieving Success at Work and In Life—One Conversation at a Time*

"Your levels of energy largely determine the quality of your life; this book shows you how to feel terrific every minute of the day!"

—Brian Tracy, author of *Change Your Thinking/Change Your Life*

"Teaches us that we can all get so much more out of our lives. I highly recommend this book to anyone who wants to be more effective, happy and energetic."

—Bruce N. Bagni, senior vice president, general counsel, Blue Cross and Blue Shield of Florida

"Jon Gordon's *Energy Addict* helps you turn your potential energy into actual energy."

—Robin Wahby, managing partner, New York Life

"Jon Gordon's strategies for boundless energy are right on target for those who want to live a full vibrant life on all levels of their being. Gordon is one of those unique individuals who lives what he teaches."

—Susan Taylor, Ph.D., author of *The Vital Energy Program*

"This is the book that people need to read right now. With so many of us needing more energy for our personal and professional lives, this clearly written, practical, and insightful book will make a powerful difference in people's lives."

—Barbara Kaufman, author of *Attitude*

"After reading *Energy Addict* I am proud to say that I am an Energy Addict. Jon Gordon's advice is concise, pertinent, and useful immediately. Changes in your life will be dramatic and will happen *right now* using his energy boosting methods. I've been recommending his energy tips to my patients with very good results. This book will get you started and his action steps will keep you energized."

—Robert Mac Murray, MD, board certified in both Family Practice (The American Board of Family Practice) and in Psychiatry and Neurology (The American Board of Psychiatry and Neurology)

"Jon is truly committed to helping others reach their full potential by tapping into their inner energy. He walks the talk! You can definitely see how very quick and simple tips have helped people change their lives. Beyond just education, I've seen employees make behavioral changes that will serve them for the long term."

—Mike Cooney, director of Human Resources, PGA Tour

"Energy is an essential ingredient in building a strong body, strong mind and strong spirit. I recommend *Energy Addict* to anyone looking to create more energy and build more strength in their life."

—Greg Finnegn, Jacksonville Jaguars and University of Colorado strength coach

ENERGY ADDICT®

101 Physical, Mental, and Spiritual Ways to Energize Your Life

JON GORDON

A Perigee Book

A Perigee Book
Published by The Berkley Publishing Group
A division of Penguin Group (USA) Inc.
375 Hudson Street
New York, New York 10014

Cover design by Ben Gibson
Cover photo by Aaron Mervin
Text design by Tiffany Estreicher

Longstreet Press hardcover edition: 2003
Perigee trade paperback edition: September 2004

Perigee trade paperback ISBN: 0-399-53089-4

Visit our website at www.penguin.com

This book has been cataloged by the Library of Congress

Printed in the United States of America

10 9 8

Contents

PART 2: MENTAL STRATEGIES

PART 3: SPIRITUAL STRATEGIES

CONCLUSION: **SHARE THE ENERGY**

ACKNOWLEDGMENTS

This book is dedicated to my wife Kathryn and my precious children. You are my teachers. Thank you for teaching me to love, play, open my heart and become a real Energy Addict. Your love, patience and support made this book possible.

To my mom and dad, thank you for always believing in me and being there with open ears and loving hearts. I am who I am because of you.

To Longstreet Press and Scott Bard, thank you for seeing my vision and helping me live my purpose.

To my brother, David Gordon, thank you for your creative ideas.

Thank you to my father for introducing me to yoga and healthy natural foods at an early age.

To my grandpa Eddy, thank you for your poems, inspiration, and example of how to live a long and healthy happy life.

I'd like to thank Arielle Ford and Brian Hilliard for believing in me and my mission. I'd like to thank Michelle Howry and John Duff for taking my vision to the next level and helping me energize even more people.

Thank you to all the people who helped me grow and share my ideas. Brian Hannafin, Ted Berkery, John Busse, Ivan Goldfarb, Richie Moran, Rick Dean, Robin Wahby, Susan Drummond, Jeff Benton, Edie Williams, Amy Waag, Rich Waag, Keith Frein, Daniel Decker, Marci Weinberg, Dave Watson, John Barry,

Ray Nealon, Matt Ray, Megan McDonough, Bob Kronmiller, Vince Bagni, Macky Weaver, Dave Donaldson, Dave Goodman, Jeffrey Harrington, Tom Carter, Becky Tokich, Tom Briones, Amy Wasserman, Elizabeth Vaeth, Tom Houck, Robert Mac Murray, MD, Susan Scott, Ken Blanchard, Michael Gerrish, Susan Taylor, Brian Tracy, Cindy Reid, Greg Finnegn, and Bruce Bagni.

INTRODUCTION

What Is an Energy Addict?

We all know someone who seems to have more energy than the rest of us. When I ask people in my seminars if they know someone who has a lot of energy, everyone in the room usually points to the same two or three people. We can see it with our eyes, hear it in their words and enthusiasm, and feel it in their presence. Just as some people are born to play the piano or baseball better than the rest of us, there are those who, I believe, are born naturally with more energy.

However, the great news is that energy can be acquired. While we may not be born as energetic as some people, we can become more energetic by acquiring more energy. Just as a baseball player can practice hitting to improve his batting skills and an actress can practice displaying different emotions to improve her craft, all of us have the ability to become skilled at acquiring more energy.

The key is to become an Energy Addict. Like any addict who is addicted to something, an Energy Addict always wants more positive energy. Energy Addicts are always interested in increasing their power supply—acquiring more energy to become more ener-

> **"The world belongs to the energetic."**
> —RALPH WALDO EMERSON

getic and powerful. If we measured an Energy Addict's energy supply it would far exceed that of a normal person. Energy Addicts take in more energy from more sources. They know where to find the energy, how to tap into it, and how to make the most of the energy they have.

Just as a good financial planner can take your $1,000 and turn it into $5,000 while an average financial planner would turn your $1,000 into $2,000, an Energy Addict can take the same amount of energy as a normal person and create more, do more and accomplish more with it. So an Energy Addict takes in more energy and makes it work more efficiently and effectively. This leads to a larger power supply even while energy is being used every day.

And because Energy Addicts are skilled at acquiring more energy for their life, they are always replacing used energy and adding to their power supply. With all of their energy, Energy Addicts also have more to share with others. This energy can be used to help other people increase their power supply—creating a more energetic company, family, organization, neighborhood and world.

As you read on, you will discover many ways to increase your power supply. Simply remember energy acquisition is a skill. The more you do it, the better you will get. The better you get, the more you will increase your power supply. You may have not been born energetic but you can become energetic. Up to this point you may have not lived a life filled with energy, but today you can become an Energy Addict.

> **"Everything is energy in motion."**
> **—PIR VILAYAT INAYAT KHAN**

How Can I Increase My Energy?

While many scientists and experts study energy, the truth is you don't have to be a scientist to know that energy is all around us and inside us. Human beings, trees, water, sunlight, air, plants and every other single thing in the universe—they're all made of energy. In fact, when we get down to it, energy is all that exists. In high school science class we learned that energy is never created nor destroyed. It is simply transformed from one form of energy to another. The energy of two cells uniting to form an embryo; a power plant turning the energy of water into electricity; a plant using the sun's energy to live—all are examples of energy flow and transformation. The same energy from sunlight that feeds an apple tree also provides us with the energy to walk, talk, and think. Energy never disappears. It is recycled into other forms of energy. Energy is never stagnant. Rather, it flows, it transforms, and it creates.

While energy is a difficult concept to grasp because we can't physically see it, we can think about our everyday experiences to understand how "it's all about energy." When we eat food, we feed our bodies energy. Sunlight and water provide a plant with the energy to live. Cars need energy to drive. When we walk into a restaurant or party, we feel the energy immediately. We instantly decide whether we like the place or we don't. We might say, "That place has great energy" or "That restaurant didn't have a good feel to it."

Likewise, we meet someone we decide immediately whether they have a "good vibe" or a "bad vibe." We read their energy and make a decision on how their energy affects us. We've all met people who have a lot of great energy. We want to be around them more. In contrast, we've also had the experience of meeting someone I call an Energy Vampire, who literally sucked the energy right out of us. If we paid close attention, we could feel the energy being pulled from our bodies. Energy Vampires do exist and they will steal your energy if you let them. I will talk about them later in the book.

Energy is also found in the thoughts we think and the words we read and hear. Have you ever gotten excited about an idea and felt energized? Or listened to an energetic speaker and become motivated to take action? Or read a book and become inspired? Words are so powerful they have started fights and wars. With each book we read and each sentence we hear, we take in energy. With each thought we think we send energy to our body and project that energy out into the world.

We also find a tremendous amount of energy in music and other people. We listen to music and it lifts us up. Have you ever seen a live concert? You can literally feel the power emanating from the performer. They are sharing their energy with the audience and the audience is receiving it. The energy is so powerful you can almost touch it.

Or have you ever been in a football or baseball stadium or basketball arena? The crowd goes wild. The home team comes from behind and wins the game. It was as if they were feeding off the energy of the crowd. They were. Or how about the way you feel after meeting an old friend for lunch or dinner. After talking to them you feel better than ever. You laughed nonstop, told stories and felt full of life. You shared energy.

Many of us also experience energy in many other ways. Have you ever said a prayer and felt God's energy fill you up? Or gone to the beach and become rejuvenated? Or hiked in the mountains and felt the energy of the trees? When you exercise do you feel like you have more energy even though you just ran two miles? When you get a good night's sleep do you feel like someone recharged your battery?

We have all of these experiences and many more like them because we are energy beings and as energy beings we interact with other forms of energy every day. We give, receive, share, transform, maximize and focus energy every day.

It's all about energy. And the key is that you can learn to create and harness energy in your own life to accomplish your goals—by becoming an Energy Addict.

The Energy Addict Lifestyle

Becoming an Energy Addict is more than just improving your physical energy. We are made up of many different types of energy—physical, mental, and spiritual. Each area of our life contributes to our total energy. Energizing only one of your energy needs is like heating only one room in your house during the winter.

Consider exercise. It may help us increase our physical and mental well-being, but it will not help us clear out negative energy from a bad relationship. This negative energy can weigh us down like a ton of bricks, no matter how much we exercise. It can cause us to be sluggish and tired even if we are in great shape. So to live a life filled with boundless energy we must address the energy needs of our parts and provide the fuel to energize the whole.

In this book I will share with you simple but powerful strategies that will increase your physical, mental and spiritual energy. These strategies are simple because anyone can do them. They can be started today. They are powerful because the small changes you make will produce big results. Many of my suggestions are backed by research and have proven themselves to be successful by all the people who use them. I have also personally incorporated the strategies, lessons and habits discussed in this book into my own life—and I continue to practice them every day. I need to. They have changed my life and I believe they will make a difference in yours.

During the past year I received many e-mails and calls from people who attended my seminars or received my "energy for life" tips via my e-mail newsletters. By incorporating one or many of my strategies into their lives, they truly found they had more energy, felt more motivated, and improved their lives significantly.

Consider Susan, who made a commitment to eat breakfast, exercise, and spend more quality time with her daughter. She is twenty pounds lighter, feels more productive at work, and now takes meaningful after-dinner walks with her daughter. They get fit together and they bond together.

Or consider Vince, who wanted to become better at focusing his energy to increase his sales. Vince's sales are up 30 percent this year because he learned how to tune out distractions and get rid of the energy vampires in his life.

Or consider Amy, who now exercises in the morning and has more energy during the day.

Brian drinks green tea in the afternoon instead of coffee and doesn't crash anymore.

And Erin is much happier since she decided to invest her energy where it matters most.

Each success story made me more inclined to share my program with as many people as possible. I believe if something works, it shouldn't be kept a secret. So I decided to write this book with the hope that it reaches those who need it the most.

For many of us, our actual energy is far below our potential energy. In fact, our energy is not even a tenth of what it could be. Yet the fact that you are reading this tells me that everything is about to change. As you read each energy tip, I am confident your actual energy will rise to meet your potential energy and the results will be amazing.

I believe positive energy is contagious. My hope is the positive energy I share with you via this book will energize your life and, in turn, you will share positive energy with others. If you find that this book helps you in your life, please tell a friend. If a strategy works for you, tell your friends so they can energize their lives. If you have a success story or lesson that you have learned, please share them with me. We are all teachers and students. While I teach the lessons I have learned, and discovered, I also continue to learn every day. Like you, I am living and working in new and changing times. As part of this process I hope you will share your thoughts and experiences with me as I share mine with you. Consider me your personal energy coach who is only a click away. You can reach me at Jon@JonGordon.com.

GIVE YOURSELF AN ENERGY AUDIT

Where do you invest your energy? How much of it is spent with meaningful people in your life? How much is spent on work? What about distractions? How about bad habits? Or goals that really don't matter anymore? Do you often relive events of the past?

I ask you to think about these questions because one of the most important things we can do to maximize our energy is to identify where we invest our energy. If 100 percent represents our total energy, then a piece of that 100 percent is invested in every person and group we spend time with. How much energy goes to people who help you become a better person?

Your Energy Audit

The Energy Audit quiz below is a way to find out where you need more energy in your life. The quiz, just like the book, is broken down into three main sections—Physical Energy, Mental Energy, and Spiritual Energy. Answer the questions below to see what

> "Too much of a good thing is wonderful."
> —MAE WEST

areas of your life are well-energized . . . and where you are in need of an energy boost.

PHYSICAL ENERGY

I wish I had more energy during the day.

- Always
- Sometimes
- Never

I hit the snooze button several times in the morning.

- Always
- Sometimes
- Never

I get less than eight hours of sleep a night.

- Always
- Sometimes
- Never

I skip breakfast.

- Always
- Sometimes
- Never

I need at least one cup of coffee to function every day.

- Always
- Sometimes
- Never

When I get to my desk, I feel exhausted before the day even begins.

- Always
- Sometimes
- Never

My energy level crashes in the afternoon.

Always Sometimes Never

I don't exercise at least three times a week.

Always Sometimes Never

I eat fast food a few times a week.

Always Sometimes Never

I feel tethered to my e-mail, voice mail, and other electronic devices.

Always Sometimes Never

If you answered "Always" or "Sometimes" to at least five of these questions, check out Part 1 to learn dozens of simple tips to bring more physical energy into your life.

MENTAL ENERGY

I feel nervous and anxious much of the time.

Always Sometimes Never

I am stressed.

Always Sometimes Never

Negative events in the news really affect me.

○ Always ○ Sometimes ○ Never

I complain.

○ Always ○ Sometimes ○ Never

I feel there is not enough time in the day.

○ Always ○ Sometimes ○ Never

Other people's actions really affect me.

○ Always ○ Sometimes ○ Never

I feel out of control when it comes to money and my finances.

○ Always ○ Sometimes ○ Never

I get into arguments with my family when I come home from work.

○ Always ○ Sometimes ○ Never

When I feel that when I finish this big project on my desk, I'll have more time to pursue the things I care about.

○ Always ○ Sometimes ○ Never

I think about events in the past and wish I acted differently.

Always Sometimes Never

If you answered "Always" or "Sometimes" to at least five of these questions, check out Part 2 to learn dozens of effective strategies to bring more mental energy into your life.

SPIRITUAL ENERGY

I feel disengaged from people around me.

Always Sometimes Never

I don't think I can really make a difference in the world.

Always Sometimes Never

I don't believe in miracles.

Always Sometimes Never

I don't have time to pray.

Always Sometimes Never

I am afraid to pursue my dreams.

Always Sometimes Never

I want to understand my purpose in life.

○ Always ○ Sometimes ○ Never

Recurring problems and struggles keep coming up in my life.

○ Always ○ Sometimes ○ Never

I am controlling and have trouble letting go.

○ Always ○ Sometimes ○ Never

If you answered "Always" or "Sometimes" to at least five of these questions, check out Part 3 to learn some smart tips to help you cultivate more spiritual energy in your life.

Invest Your Energy in What Matters Most

Once you decide where you are currently investing your energy, the next step is to decide what changes need to be made. What should be discarded and what in your life should receive more of your energy? A strategy I use during this process is to ask energy questions. Does this person increase my energy or zap my energy? Does a certain organization or business group increase my energy or drain my energy? Does it increase my business or simply take up my time? And the single most important question I ask is, am I investing my energy in what matters most? Does my continued investment in this person, group, belief, and habit make me a better person? Will it matter a year or two from now? Does it improve society and those closest to me? The answers will help you direct your energy where it should be spent.

> **"Life begets energy. Energy creates energy. It is only by spending oneself wisely that one becomes rich in life."**
> **—ELEANOR ROOSEVELT**

When possible, the things in your life that drain your energy or don't really matter should receive a minute amount of your energy. Negative feelings about a person in the past should be let go so you can invest your energy to create your present and future. People who waste your time and energy should be replaced with those who enrich your life. Remember, for each of us, what matters most and what enriches us will be different. The key is to know what matters most to you and learn to invest a majority of your energy on these priorities.

When you invest your energy in what matters most you receive the biggest return on your investments. You use your energy to develop and create what you value most. Instead of knocking your building down you build it with one positive investment at a time. If you invest more time with your children you will see their growth immediately. If you invest in positive beliefs instead of negative thoughts you will create an annuity of positive events and people in your life. If you tune out distractions and spend more time where it matters most you will be more productive and successful in whatever you do. Investing your energy in what matters most will be the best investment you have ever made.

Put Your Own Energy First

Imagine you're an energy vending machine. Your family comes up to you, puts a few coins in and says, "We need some energy!"

Do you have any to give? Or are you already spent? Are you stocked up or sold out? Or think about your boss standing by your machine. Now that's a scary thought. He is looking at you deciding if he wants a large or a small amount of energy today. Do you have the energy to give?

There are a lot of people looking to put coins in us and if we don't have the energy to give, they'll likely bang on the machine looking for their money back. Let's just hope they don't tip the machine over. The fact is, we can't give what we don't have. To give energy we need to have energy. To have energy we need to put our energy first. This means that we need to stock up our vending machine before we give it to everyone else. While some may call this selfish, I call it smart. While some may call you self-centered, I call you generous. If you put your energy first you will have more energy for yourself and more to share with others.

Consider Ted. Ted is always giving to everyone. He ignores his own needs, works tirelessly, gets little sleep and spends his free time making sure everyone else is happy. Everyone else receives his energy but Ted has nothing left for himself. Everyone says, "WOW, look at how giving Ted is. Isn't he great?" But Ted's machine becomes empty. In the future Ted may burn out. Or Ted will likely get sick and will not be there for his family when they need him. Or Ted might leave his family to find so-called "happiness."

Now consider Ed. Ed puts his energy first. Ed stocks up on energy. Ed makes time for exercise, sleep, play and himself. Ed takes care of himself so he has something left to give his family. Ed takes care of himself so he has more energy for his career. Ed knows that he can't give his energy if he doesn't have any for himself. In the end everyone in Ed's life is better off because Ed put his energy first.

So remember, even when society criticizes you for putting

your energy first, be like Ed. This doesn't mean you are selfish. You put your energy first and then you share your energy with others. You get a massage so you will be more relaxed during the week. If you are a mom with small children, you hire that sitter for a few hours so you can recharge and rejuvenate. You take your lunch break in the park so you can be more productive in the afternoon. You exercise in the morning so you can spend time with your kids in the evening. You ask your husband or wife to watch the kids so you can take some time for yourself. You balance your personal life and career. In the long run everyone you live with, work with and interact with will thank you. Those who have the energy are the ones who can share it. Instead of handing out your energy to everyone else remember to first stock up your energy vending machine and then you can dispense your energy accordingly. When those who need you most put their quarters in, you'll have plenty of energy to give.

Combine Strategies for Energy Building

As you get further into this book, you'll find several strategies that, when done together, will increase your energy exponentially. I call this practice "energy building," because you build your life with one energy source at a time that when added together make a big difference. Like a ladder, consider each new habit as a rung that will take your energy one step higher.

Energy building is all about selecting a few of the tips suggested in this book and incorporating them into your life one at a time. As you add each habit to your life you will see your energy increase higher and higher. The key is to take small steps rather than trying to do too much at once. We don't want anyone to create an energy overload and blow out their power plant. Make one or at most a few tips a habit at a time and then add another energy tip. With each action you will build your life and increase your energy.

Energy building can be done with various energy sources. Exercising in the morning (page 50), eating breakfast (page 25), and starting your day with positive thoughts (page 99) will help you create a more energetic and productive morning. Eating a snack before dinner (page 31), eating a light and healthy dinner (page 23), and walking after lunch (page 52) will fuel your night with more energy, more fun and happiness. Remember, you don't need to do everything in this book. Simply decide what works for you, practice energy building, and watch your energy soar.

One of my clients simply put three of my tips into practice and lost weight, noticed increased energy, and became a motivator to her employees and family. My client and her daughter now take after-dinner walks allowing them to spend more time together and live more energetically.

Create Rituals That Will Become Your Foundation

As part of any "energy for life" plan, rituals are the key to turning our goals into reality—or chaos into concrete action. Rituals help us create positive habits that will become our foundation in a crazy world.

For example, when I was at the peak of my unhappiness several years ago I asked myself what was missing in my life. The answers were loud and clear—a healthy diet, exercise, creative expression, and time with my wife and kids. So I developed my

> **"The most accomplished performers have defined specific rituals in daily life where as those who are less successful do not."**
> **—JAMES E. LOEHR, ED.D, AUTHOR AND PSYCHOLOGIST**

routine and rituals around those very things. My wife and I decided to make Saturday night our date night; every Saturday we would hire a babysitter and go out for dinner and a movie. I started writing every night after I read to my daughter and put her down to sleep. It became a priority to get home each night so that I could spend time with her before she went to bed.

On the exercise and diet front I created exercise routines and diets and made them a part of my everyday life. I went to the same deli every morning and ordered four egg whites and fruit for breakfast before heading into work. I liked walking in the door and holding four fingers in the air; the cooks knew what to make. Amazingly, these routines and rituals helped bring a certain order and peace to my life that made everything flow much easier. My habits became my life and I was much happier.

By incorporating meaningful habits into our lives with rituals and routines, we make our lives more meaningful. This gives us a foundation and a center that we can build on and around. We can develop a routine or ritual for anything. Perhaps we walk our dog every night before we go to bed. Or we do yoga before we shower in the morning. We eat French toast every Sunday. We call our special friends once a month at the same time. If we are single, we might go to a social event once a week every Thursday. If we are married, we might call our spouse every day at noon to ask how he or she is doing. If we are religious, we most likely go to a religious service once a week. If we are spiritual, we likely meditate and pray daily.

Our life is the result of our words, choices, thoughts and actions. What we believe, say, choose and do is what we become. When you create rituals that increase your mental, physical and spiritual energy, you become more energetic, happier and successful.

As you read more of this book, write down the strategies that you want to incorporate into your life and decide what ritual will help you make it a habit. Use my action steps at the end of each section as a guide and decide the best times and days to incorporate each power source in your life.

Use my ritual planner below as a guide. You can easily recreate this ritual planner on a separate sheet of paper.

Strategy: Eat a healthy breakfast before work

Action: Eat breakfast

Time: 7am

Days: Monday–Friday

Complete the ritual contract below and tape this to your mirror and carry a copy in your car. Also add this ritual schedule to your daily planner or calendar.

I will incorporate ______________________ **into my life**

strategy

by ______________________________________

doing what

at ________________ **on** ____________________

time *day(s)*

Your contract might look something like:

I will incorporate a healthy breakfast into my life by eating breakfast at 7am, Monday through Friday.

Signature ____

PART 1

PHYSICAL STRATEGIES

1

Value Your Body

How much do you value your body? What is it worth to you? Ask a person in need of an organ transplant, and they would say that a healthy body is priceless. Ask a scientist or doctor, and they would tell you "millions of dollars." But if we are worth so much, then why do so many of us value our body so little?

Unfortunately many of us take better care of our $20,000 cars than our priceless body. We don't exercise our million-dollar body because we have to work fifteen hours a day at our $60,000 a year job. We allow everything else to be more important than our health—and then we wonder why we get sick, gain weight, lose sleep, and get depressed. In fact, we often don't value our body or treat it with respect until *after* we have caused ourselves serious harm, or are in danger from diseases such as cancer or heart disease. Only when our health is threatened do we put a significant value on it. Only when we are in danger of losing our health do we treasure it.

The good news is things can change. Values can change. Actions can change. Today we can begin to value our body more than we value anything else. We can invest our energy in our body and our health. No matter how busy we are, a short walk each day will pay incredible dividends. Eating more fruits, vegetables, and whole

> **"If you have your health, you truly have everything."**
> **—JANICE GORDON**

grains will add years to our lives. Recharging your batteries each night with at least eight hours of sleep will make you operate optimally.

Our health is certainly more valuable than any mutual fund, any job, or any project. And when you value your body more than anything else, you will actually create more success in all the areas of your life. One of my grandmother's favorite sayings was, "if you have your health you have everything." I agree—when you value your body, your investment will provide you with everything you need for as long as you have it.

ACTION STEPS

1. Write the following words on a piece of paper and carry it in your calendar, your date book, or your checkbook: "My body is worth millions of dollars."

2. Carry this paper with you in your pocket and look at it once a day. Remind yourself to invest your energy in your health before you invest in anything else.

2

Feed Your Body Life

Today more than ever, we need to fuel our bodies with the best sources of energy. We need to eat real foods that fuel our passion, our drive, and our busy schedule. We need to feed our body life. To do this, I recommend that you eat whole foods whenever possible.

What are "whole foods"? Whole foods are foods that have not been processed—foods from nature. They have a short shelf life and usually contain just one or two ingredients. Several examples of whole foods include raisins, nuts, apples, beans, rice, spinach, salmon, eggs, lean meats, and bananas.

Whole foods differ from the processed foods that make up much of our modern diet. Processed foods can sit on a shelf a long time, contain 5 or more ingredients made up of multisyllabic words we can't pronounce, and often contain partially hydrogenated oils and preservatives to give them a longer shelf life. Look on any supermarket shelf and you'll find mostly processed foods.

The simple fact is that our natural bodies perform best when fed natural foods. Just as a car engine needs high quality fuel to run properly we need high quality energy to ensure peak performance. Foods from nature contain the most and best sources of energy, whereas most processed foods are made up of empty calories with little energy or benefit to us. While it is difficult to make whole foods 100 percent of your diet, there are some simple ways to start to incorporate them into your menu. We'll talk about some specific ways in the next several pages. While there is much confusing and conflicting information and research regarding the best diets to lose weight, the research is clear—if we eat more fresh vegetables, fruits, whole grains, and lean sources of protein we increase our chances of living longer, healthier, more energetic lives. No matter what diet you may be on in the short run, remember that in the long run our bodies do best when fed nature's energy. To help you incorporate high-energy sources of fuel into your life try the following simple action steps. You will feel the difference.

ACTION STEPS

1. Think of food as fuel. Eat foods closest to nature so you build your body every day with the best sources of energy.

2. When choosing your foods, read the labels and know what you're putting into your body. For example, Smucker's Natural Peanut Butter is made with just peanuts and salt. That's it. Wow—what a concept.

3. Reduce the amount of processed foods in your diet.

3

Visit a Health Food Store

This strategy will only take an hour—but if you have never been to a health food store, the experience will open your eyes to a new and healthy world full of great energy. When I lived in Atlanta, I remember my first visit to a health food store called Return2Eden. I found a whole array of products that were similar to the ones I would buy in a regular supermarket . . . but more natural and healthier. Sure, many of these products are a little more expensive, but with the popularity of stores such as Whole Foods Market and the creation of entire health sections in regular supermarkets, it is becoming even easier to find large selections of organic and natural foods at decent prices.

The people who work at these health food stores are great resources themselves—they can explain what makes certain products better than others and recommend the best vitamins to fit your needs. Visiting these stores will also teach you to read the ingredients of everything you buy and help you become more conscious of the food you are feeding your body. You will become more educated and empowered to make better choices for your health and energy.

A surprising side effect of eating from a health-food store: many of the snacks there actually taste a lot *better* than the foods found at a regular supermarket. For example, I now eat Fig Newmans instead of Fig Newtons. Read the ingredients and you'll see a big difference. I eat Smuckers Natural Peanut Butter with no hydrogenated oil instead of Jiff or Skippy (both of which contain corn syrup and hydrogenated oil). And I eat all-natural cheese instead of processed cheese loaded with chemicals. Give it a try and see how healthy (and tasty) this food can be.

ACTION STEP

Take a visit to a health food store or a mega health food store such as Whole Foods. Walk the aisles. Ask questions. Try a few products that sound interesting, and compare them to the versions you're used to eating in your regular supermarket. See what a difference the healthier food makes in your energy level.

4

Eat More Earlier

One of the simple keys to increased energy is to eat a majority of your calories earlier in the day rather than later in the evening. According to one preliminary study, Dr. R. Curtis Ellison at Boston University School of Medicine showed that, compared to French men and women, who consume 57 percent of their daily calories before 2:00 pm and are very active in the evening, Americans take in only 38 percent of their daily calories before 2:00 pm. And as many of us know, many Americans eat a large dinner before stumbling over to the couch to watch television until bedtime.

> **"Eat breakfast like a king, lunch like a prince and dinner like a college kid with a maxed out charge card."**
>
> **—JON GORDON**

So what effect does eating a majority of our calories earlier in the day have on our bodies and energy? According to Dr. Robert K. Cooper, author of *High Energy Living*, in a study conducted at the University of Minnesota, researchers compared groups of people on 2,000-calorie-a-day diets to find out which groups had the most energy and lost the most weight. The study showed people who ate their 2,000 calories earlier in the day had the most energy and lost weight—an average of 2.3 pounds per week. People *who ate the same amount of calories* but who consumed most of those calories later in the day actually gained weight and felt more tired.

To help you eat more calories earlier in the day, here are a few Action Steps. Some of these Action Steps are so important they deserve their own strategy.

ACTION STEPS

1. Eat a healthy and satisfying breakfast.
2. Eat energizing snacks throughout the day for increased energy.
3. Try not to eat dinner past 7 pm. Ideally try to eat before 6 pm.
4. Eat smaller meals but more of them. Instead of two or three large meals eat three meals and two snacks.
5. On weekends, eat your main meal at midday.

5

Eat Breakfast

Many of us think that if we want to lose weight then we should skip breakfast. After all, if we don't eat breakfast that means we're consuming fewer calories. Right?

Ironically, one of the keys to losing weight and increasing your metabolism is to eat a hearty and healthy breakfast. And one of the simplest things you can do to increase your energy during the day is to eat breakfast.

When you eat breakfast you activate your body's "thermal switch," which helps you burn fat and produce energy throughout the day. Studies show if you eat breakfast you are more alert and you perform better at work. Breakfast eaters also show less fatigue and are usually leaner than those who skip breakfast.

According to Dr. Sarah Leibiwitz of Rockefeller University in New York City, when you skip breakfast you are also more likely to gorge on high fat, high sugar foods at night. Many of us can attest to this in our own struggles with gaining and losing weight. If we skip meals throughout the day, we often lose control when it's finally time to eat. Instead of gulping a cup of coffee and running out the door, make time for a quick and healthy breakfast.

ACTION STEPS

1. Plan. Decide what you are going to eat for breakfast the night before, so when you wake up tired and sluggish you already have a clear plan of action.

2. Make it healthy. Pop-Tarts and high sugar cereals don't count. You might as well eat a candy bar. Instead, eat foods high in fiber, high in protein, and low in fat. Several examples of a great breakfast:

    - Oatmeal with low-fat milk and a piece of fruit
    - Three eggs, a piece of fruit, and a slice of whole-grain bread
    - A bowl of low-fat plain yogurt mixed with low-fat granola, a cut-up banana, and raisins
    - Whole-grain toast with Smucker's Natural Peanut Butter

3. Make time for breakfast. Get up ten minutes earlier. Think of it this way: a few minutes to eat breakfast will give you hours of increased energy and productivity. It's worth it.

6

Cut the Caffeine

Too often I see people pumping Mountain Dew, coffee, soda and energy drinks into their mouths as they look for a quick buzz and a jolt of energy to help them work harder and faster. When the caffeine high wears off, they guzzle another one or grab a candy bar for a sugar high. Others drink coffee after coffee.

Yes, in the short run this may work. The caffeine and sugar may give you a quick boost of energy. But like any drug, they wear off . . . and to keep the high going you need more and more and more. The problem is, when you rely on caffeine and sugar for energy instead of healthy foods you are setting yourself up for fatigue and burnout.

According to Dr. Andrew Weil, author of *8 Weeks to Optimum Health*, sugar has strong druglike effects in some people. Sugar can give you a rush of energy, followed by a metabolic crash soon after. He says, "This cycle is extremely disruptive to the body's energy cycle and can trigger disturbing mood swings." And caffeine may stimulate stress hormones that give you temporary energy but also affect your natural energy cycle. Excessive caffeine and sugar give you the appearance they are supplying you with energy but in reality they drain the life out of you. The old adage "what goes up, must come down," rings true. While caffeine and sugar may take your energy sky high, they also cause it to come crashing down.

To stop the crashing you have to keep filling your body with these energy sources and so begins the process I call a vicious cycle. I see it all the time as I travel around the country. Instead of eating food, drinking water and getting enough sleep people try to stay energized with caffeine. People wonder why they don't have any energy. They wonder why they are always tired and I believe relying on caffeine instead of food, sleep and water for energy is one of the main reasons. They are living on short bursts, quick fixes and a bunch of bull instead of the real power sources that will provide them with fuel for life.

ACTION STEPS

1. Chose water or green tea instead of soda or coffee.
2. Drink sparkling water instead of soda if you want some bubbles.
3. Buy a water filter for your home to drink the best water possible.
4. When choosing bottled water, try to buy purified water.

7

Drink Green Tea

I am a big fan of green tea, and I promote its benefits whenever I speak. I love hearing from all the people who share with me how green tea has improved their health and enhanced their energy.

While all "real" tea comes from the same plant Camellia sinensis, the benefits of green tea result because of the way the leaves are processed. I first learned about the benefits of green tea from my favorite health and wellness expert, Dr. Andrew Weil. According to Dr. Weil, green tea is prepared in a much more gentle fashion than ordinary black tea—the green tea leaves are steamed, rolled and dried (rather than crushed), a method that preserves the antioxidant compounds that give us health benefits. Dr. Weil states these antioxidants protect our heart by lowering cholesterol and improving lipid metabolism, and guard against cancer by scavenging for free radicals that can damage cells and push them in the direction of uncontrolled growth. Green tea also has antibacterial effects. The Chinese have been drinking green tea for years and now numerous studies are reporting that green tea helps us fight against cancer and prevent heart disease.

But there is more to the green tea story. In addition to the health benefits of green tea, I drink it and recommend it because it is a great alternative to coffee and caffeinated energy drinks. Green tea contains anywhere from 26 mg to 40 mg of caffeine, about half or one-third the amount of coffee. Like coffee, it gives you an energy boost to kick-start your day or wake you up in the afternoon. Yet because it doesn't contain as much caffeine, green tea doesn't take you as high as coffee and doesn't cause you to crash afterward. The effects of green tea feel more like an energy boost than an energy jolt.

ACTION STEPS

1. Try drinking a cup of green tea in the morning. You can drink it hot, or you can drink it cold by cooling it in your refrigerator or pouring it over ice.

2. Drink green tea instead of coffee, caffeinated sodas, and energy drinks.

3. If you are a big fan of your morning coffee (like my wife is!), then have your coffee in the morning but replace your afternoon cup of coffee with a cup of green tea.

Note: If you must stay away from caffeine for medical reasons, decaffeinated green tea is also available and provides your body with antioxidants. When choosing a decaffeinated green tea, select a brand that is naturally decaffeinated without chemicals.

8

Grab a Snack

Just as we need to constantly feed a fire with moderate size pieces of wood, we also need to continually supply our internal furnace with food that can be turned into fuel. This keeps our metabolism going strong and steady.

Research published in the *New England Journal of Medicine* recommends that we will benefit greatly if we eat smaller, more frequent meals and spread out our food intake throughout the day rather than eating one or two large meals. According to Dr. Dan Benardot at Georgia State University in Atlanta, we should eat every three hours or so to stay satiated and energized. Studies show if you have moderate-size meals plus small between-meal snacks, you increase your levels of energy and alertness. Without healthy snacks, your blood sugar falls and you experience fatigue and tension.

Eating smaller, more frequent meals pushes our energy higher and keeps our mind sharper. With a constant supply of fuel for our mind and body, our memory is enhanced, we learn more, and our performance excels. The keys are to choose healthy smaller meals and eat energizing snacks. Here are a few of my favorite energy snacks:

- A smoothie made with fresh fruit, yogurt, and ice
- A handful of raisins and nuts
- Whole-grain bread with a piece of cheese

- A protein shake
- Vegetarian chili or soup
- A piece of fruit
- Whole-wheat cracker with a little peanut butter
- Hummus, pita bread and vegetables

ACTION STEPS

1. Plan your meal and snacks the night before.

2. When you are traveling or are driving around bring healthy snacks with you or else when you become hungry you will likely run into a convenience store and grab a bag of chips.

9

Don't Skip Lunch

It's a popular notion that we will get more done if we skip lunch. Today hundreds of thousands of people will skip lunch in order to accomplish more at work: "I have too much to do. I can't make lunch today." "Lunch is a waste of time. I'll tough it out and get more done." "I'm swamped. No time for lunch." I know—I used to buy into this belief as well.

Unfortunately this couldn't be further from the truth. Dr. Etienne Grandjean, an expert on productivity at the Swiss Federal Institute of Technology, says eating a good lunch is highly recommended "for both health and work efficiency." According to various studies, researchers agree that performance scores plunge when people skip lunch, and found that those who skip lunch soon feel more anxious and tense. Skipping lunch can also slow your metabolism and cut your energy production throughout the day . . . leading to a ravenous appetite at dinnertime.

Ironically, the desire to get ahead and get more done actually leads to *less* productivity and burn-out if lunch is skipped on a regular basis. People will often try to compensate for their lack of energy by drinking coffee or caffeinated drinks instead of eating lunch. However, this simply makes a bad mistake worse by causing your body and brain to work harder and harder on less fuel. Our bodies need to recharge with a relaxing lunch break and a satisfying lunch, and instead we're making our motors work beyond capacity. Eventually our motors will burn out.

Think of it this way. A 20-minute lunch will provide you with hours of energy. It's worth it.

ACTION STEPS

1. Plan your meals the night before. Experts say that we make between 20 and 30 food choices a day. If we make these choices when we are so hungry, we can't even think we are more likely to go through the fast-food drive-thru than eating a healthy lunch.

2. Don't overeat. There's nothing worse than eating a huge lunch and then feeling horrible the rest of the day . . . especially if you're stuck behind a desk with nowhere to "walk it off." The key is to eat a big enough lunch to satisfy you but not so big that you need a nap afterward. If you find yourself getting filled up, ask for a to-go box and eat the rest as a mid-afternoon snack.

3. Eat protein. Nutrition experts recommend we include some protein as part of our lunch. Proteins such as turkey, chicken, fish, and lean meat take longer to digest which sustains our blood sugar level and keeps us from being hungry again soon after lunch.

4. Remember to eat whole foods. No matter what diet you may be trying, the best source of fuel for our body and brain are foods from nature. Instead of white processed bread choose whole-grain bread. Instead of fat-filled processed foods, choose whole grains, beans, legumes, fruits, and vegetables.

10

Drink Water to Survive and Thrive

One of the simplest and most powerful things you can do to energize your life is to drink water. Our bodies are constantly losing water, and studies show that a decrease in water consumption leads to fatigue and headaches. Since our bodies are mostly made of water, our bodies and brains work best when they are fully hydrated. Water helps deliver important nutrients, energy, and messages to the various cells in our bodies. Water is the fuel our bodies and brains need to survive and thrive. Just as oil helps a car engine function optimally, water helps us operate at peak performance. And the best thing about water is you can find it everywhere.

ACTION STEPS

1. Most experts agree that the average person needs to drink six to eight cups of water every day to stay healthy. If you exercise you will likely need even more.

2. Rather than drinking your daily allowance of water all at once, try to consume small amounts of water every 30 minutes during the day. This will keep you energized and alert all day long.

3 While water is better than soda, there are also brands of water that are better than others. Check out Penta Water at www.Pentawater.com. If water were gas, Penta Water would be considered high-octane fuel.

11

Sip Small Amounts of Chilled Water Every 30 Minutes

Try it now and see how this simple habit refreshes and energizes you.

Studies show that when you consume small amounts of chilled water every 20–30 minutes during the day, you provide a strong, clear, and continual signal to your body to keep your energy elevated. In addition, you improve your overall health and resistance to illness. While it is not yet a scientific fact, studies by Dr. Darden, the director of research for Nautilus Sports/Medical Industries in Colorado Springs, suggest that you get even more energized by drinking ice-cold water than water at room temperature. He says, "A gallon of ice-cold water requires more than 200 calories of heat energy to warm it to the core body temperature of 98.6 degrees." Thus, this heat energy that your body creates to warm the cold water provides you with more energy for your life.

Another reason to sip water every 30 minutes is to keep your kidneys fully hydrated. If your kidneys do not get enough water, function is hindered, waste products accumulate, and the liver assumes the role of flushing out the impurities. This diverts the liver from its main duty of metabolizing stored fat into usable energy. This means less burning of your body fat and less energy for you. This also explains one of the reasons why drinking plenty of water helps you lose weight and body fat.

Human beings lose about nine cups of water a day through breathing, perspiration, urination, and bowel movements. And this doesn't include water loss through physical exercise, which results in even more water loss. When you sip chilled water every 30 minutes you replenish your water loss and provide your body with more energy for life. Try it now and feel the energy difference.

ACTION STEPS

1. **Befriend a cup or bottle of cold water. If you work at home, keep one in the refrigerator.**

2. **If you work in an office keep a bottle of water cold with an insulator. Or even bring a mini-cooler of ice with you to work.**

3. **Sip the water every 30 minutes and energize your body and brain.**

12

Get Nuts

Eat almonds, pumpkin seeds and walnuts. I try to eat a handful a day. They are a great source of energy and healthy fat. Many people protest: "I can't eat nuts, they're fattening." The truth is, nuts are only fattening if you eat the entire jar or bag. Research tells us we need to eat good sources of fat to burn fat. Grab a handful and put the rest away.

Another healthy source of "good fat" is flaxseed. Incorporate flaxseeds into your diet—it's a great sources of omega-3 essential fatty acids. Sprinkle ground flaxseeds on your cereal or oatmeal. You can buy flaxseeds in your local health food store or Whole Foods Market.

ACTION STEPS

1. **Instead of chips and candy bars, eat a handful of nuts or raisins as a snack.**
2. **Grind some flaxseed and sprinkle it over your cereal tomorrow morning.**

13

Soup Up Your Life

Growing up in a Jewish-Italian family, chicken soup was a big part of my childhood. As soon as one of us became sick with a cold or fever, Mom made a pot of chicken soup . . . and we always felt better. Well, now we know that chicken soup does more than nourish the body and soul. Researchers at Johns Hopkins University in Baltimore discovered that chicken soup and other soups increase our energy—while also reducing fat cravings. The research showed that people ate significantly less during their meals if they had soup beforehand. Furthermore, out of many different appetizers, soup was considered the most satisfying and invigorating.

While this kind of scientific research is helpful, we also know from our personal experience that a healthy soup gives us energy. As a child, I remember coming into the house after playing football and eating a bowl of soup. It always rejuvenated me. How does soup make you feel? After a hearty and healthy bowl do you feel energized? If so, try to eat soup more often for more energy. Note that not all soups are created equally. When it comes to eating food for energy, avoid beef-base, pork-base, and cream-base soups.

ACTION STEPS

1. Visit your local health food store or the health food section of your supermarket and notice the different brands and types of soup. These soups are made with natural ingredients and often less sodium.

2. If you work in an office, bring your soup in a container or bowl and eat it as a snack to keep you going until lunch, or eat it during lunch with a salad or sandwich.

3. Eat soup before dinner as an appetizer and eat a light energizing dinner.

4. Each week, make a big batch of soup and keep it in the refrigerator. When you get hungry, just soup it up.

5. Check out various soup books, such as *Saved by Soup: More Than 100 Delicious Low-Fat Soup Recipes to Eat and Enjoy Every Day* by Judith Barrett.

6. Visit www.souprecipe.com for hundreds of other great soup recipes.

14

Replace Your Candy Bowl with a Fruit Bowl

If you walk into your office or home and see a bowl of candy, your first instinct is to grab a piece. Why not? After all, it's sitting right there, calling our names. I used to work in an office where candy and chocolate could be found on just about everyone's desk. When someone became hungry, he had a candy bar. By the end of the day, we'd be sluggish and grumpy. Does this sound like your office?

By having a candy bowl so easily available, it literally takes a tremendous amount of energy *not* to eat it on a regular basis. The same goes for our homes. If we keep a candy bowl on the kitchen counter, sure enough we'll grab for it every time. Thankfully there is a simple solution to this problem. Make the switch.

Replace your candy bowl in your office or home with a fruit bowl. You'll not only increase your energy, but you'll also energize your co-workers or family members. At first they may grumble. But once they see the difference a healthy pick-me-up makes in the way they feel, you'll start to find some converts. And, most of all, a fruit bowl on your desk or in your home will help you make healthy food choices. When hunger sets in, your impulse will be to reach for an apple instead of running for the vending machine.

ACTION STEPS

1. Buy a decent size bowl for your home, and each week replenish it with fresh fruit.

2. If you work in an office, buy a bowl for your desk and fill it up with fresh fruit. If other people often eat your fruit, start a "fruit fund" and you can buy fruit for them also.

3. If you work in an office, ask your HR person if the company would support a fruit bowl in the break room.

4. At home, talk to your family and explain to them why you have made the switch from the candy bowl to a fruit bowl.

15

Trash the Hydrogenated Oils

If you read the ingredients on most of the products found in supermarkets you will see the words, "partially hydrogenated" or "hydrogenated oil." Hydrogenated oil is found in almost every prepared food, including margarine, shortening (i.e., Crisco), breads, crackers, cookies, soups, sauces, frozen meals, desserts and chips. Unfortunately for us, putting hydrogenated oils into your body is like putting tar into your veins or sludge into a car's engine.

Think of your body as an energy machine, made up of 100 trillion energy cells. When you fuel those cells with bad oil, you get less output and have less energy. When you feed your cells good oils, such as olive oil, you ensure peak performance. Bad oil = bad energy. Great oil = great energy.

Through the hydrogenation process, hydrogen is heated and pumped into liquid unsaturated oil in order to solidify it and give it a longer shelf life. This process of heating oil to solidify it produces trans fatty acids (TFAs), which are very harmful to our bodies. Clinical studies have shown that trans-fat raises LDL cholesterol levels (the bad cholesterol) while lowering the HDL levels (the good cholesterol in your body)—increasing your risk of coronary heart disease.

Increasing awareness about the health hazards of TFAs and hydrogenated oils are even causing major food companies to make changes. In fact, Frito-Lay now offers trans fat-free Doritos, Cheetos, and Tostitos. They use expeller pressed oil as opposed to partially hydrogenated soybean oil. But until more large food manufacturers make changes, we have to make changes ourselves.

Here are a few ways to trash the hydrogenated oils.

ACTION STEPS

1. Check the labels and ingredients of any processed foods you buy and avoid those containing hydrogenated or partially hydrogenated oils of any kind.

2. Buy snacks, breads, crackers, soups and many other products from your local health food store, the health food section of your supermarket or from a store such as Whole Foods. Many of these stores will have products that contain expeller-pressed organic oils instead of hydrogenated oils.

3. Avoid fast-food restaurants unless you know they use healthy oils.

4. Remember one of my favorite sayings from Dr. Weil—manufacturers hydrogenate oil to give products a longer shelf life . . . however, a longer shelf life for them means a shorter shelf life for you.

16

Practice the 90-10 Rule

I was having dessert in a restaurant once with my wife when a person recognized me from one of my Energy Addict seminars. He approached us and said, "Hey, you're the energy guy." Then he looked at my plate and frowned. "You can't be eating dessert!"

We all laughed, and I had to explain my 90-10 rule. The two fundamental principles of the 90-10 rule are: 1) We should eat healthy, energizing, natural food 90 percent of the time; and 2) we all deserve to treat ourselves. I am a firm believer that if we deprive ourselves of our favorite treats—such as ice cream, desserts, donuts, candy—then our lives as Energy Addicts will never feel natural or sustained. It's like a diet that says you can only eat meat, or an exercise program that says you have to work out in a gym five days a week. At some point it will be difficult to maintain these programs and diets because they don't flow with our natural lifestyles and rhythms. They feel forced, and once we stop them we revert back to our old habits. The best programs and the best diets help people incorporate lifelong habits into their lives. Instead of a diet or program, these habits become who we are. They become our way of life.

You can be an Energy Addict without depriving yourself. You know you fuel your body with the best fuel 90 percent of the time . . . and 10 percent of the time you treat yourself and satisfy your cravings. Next time we happen to see each other eating dessert in a restaurant, we'll nod at each other, smile, and know the 90-10 rule is in effect!

ACTION STEPS

1. When you first start eating healthier, energizing foods, plan a treat three times a week. Once on Monday, once on Wednesday and once on Friday. You are in the habit-forming stage at this point and thus structure is important.

2. After a month, scale back your treats to 2 times a week.

3. After you feel like eating healthy energizing meals and snacks has truly become a comfortable habit, then you should eat treats 10 percent of the time, whenever the situation or desire presents itself. Trust me, eating energizing food 90 percent of the time will actually make you *not* want to eat treats that often—once you eat sugary foods, you'll feel their negative effects immediately.

17

Be Active

When we think of exercise, we often think of putting on our exercise clothes, stretching, raising our heart rates, and sweating like crazy. However, there are many great ways to energize our mind and bodies that don't take a lot of time and don't require a lot of planning. These activities help you BE ACTIVE. They get your body in motion. They make you move a little more and get the energy circulating through your body. Our bodies were not meant to sit at desks and couches all day. They were meant to walk, move, run, and be active. While many of us don't have a choice of what we do on company time, we do have a choice to be active on our time. Here are a few Action Steps to help you choose to BE ACTIVE.

> **"If not now, when?"**
> **—THE TALMUD**

ACTION STEPS

1. **Take the stairs at work instead of the elevator.**
2. **Park in the farthest row from the grocery store.**
3. **Take a short walk after lunch and dinner.**

4. Instead of letting your dog hang out in the backyard take her for a walk.

5. If it's not far away, ride your bike to the grocery store for a few needed items.

6. Walk and talk with your kids or grandkids after dinner.

7. Stand up and stretch throughout the day.

8. Do some yard work.

9. Help clean up the house.

10. Put on some music and dance by yourself or with your significant other.

18

Exercise in the Morning

When people ask me the best time to exercise, I recommend the morning. When you exercise in the morning, your body and brain work together to kick-start your metabolism. Your brain tells your body, "Hey, we are going to be busy today, start producing some energy." Your body kicks in and starts burning fuel to provide the energy your brain says it needs. This helps increase your energy production and alertness.

Another benefit of morning exercise is that it is easier to make exercise a habit when we do it in the morning. If we wait until lunch or the end of the day, it's more likely we'll feel too tired or other obstacles will get in the way. According to Robert Cooper, Ph.D., a study by the Southwestern Health Institute in Phoenix found that three out of four people who did some light morning exercise continued the exercise habit one year later. In comparison, only half of those who waited until midday to exercise were able to keep up the habit. And among those who said, "I'll do it in the evening," only one out of every four were still exercising a year after the study began.

"A journey of a thousand miles begins with a single step."
—CONFUCIUS

ACTION STEPS

1. Plan your exercise the night before. Lay out your exercise clothes on your dresser. This will help remind you of your commitment.

2. Do one form of light exercise. You can take a walk around your neighborhood. Walk up and down your stairs. Play and follow a yoga video. Do push-ups or abdominal stretches. If you have a stationary bike read the paper or a book while you pedal. Watch television while you walk on a treadmill. Remember, you don't need a gym or expensive equipment. All you need is a pair of shoes and a place to walk.

3. Visit www.jorgecruise.com for simple exercises that only take eight minutes in the morning, and read Jorge's book *8 Minutes in the Morning*.

19

Take a Walk After Lunch

Do you often feel like collapsing into a big chair and taking a nap after lunch? You sit at your desk or on your couch at home trying to fight the urge to fall asleep. You feel as unproductive as a plumber without a wrench. There is a solution—walking for five to ten minutes after lunch can greatly increase our energy for the rest of the day. While eating a healthy moderate-sized lunch will give us energy, walking after lunch will multiply the energy-boosting effect of food. When we exercise after lunch we burn even more calories and produce even more energy for our body.

Robert E. Thayer, Ph. D., professor of biological psychology at California State University, found that as little as 10 minutes of brisk walking leads to very significant increases in energy. Even a light walk energizes me and helps me be more productive after lunch and throughout the afternoon. I continue the practice to this day. While I often become hungry sooner (because of the increase in calories and fuel I'm burning), I simply eat an energizing snack, which keeps me even more alert until dinner. Just try it for a few weeks, and you'll find out for yourself.

> **"The higher your energy level, the more efficient your body. The more efficient your body, the better you feel and the more you will use your talent to produce outstanding results."**
>
> —ANTHONY ROBBINS

ACTION STEPS

1. If you drive to lunch, park far enough away from the restaurant so you have to take a light walk to and from your car.

2. If your office is near restaurants, walk to and from lunch. Or drive with a friend and walk back.

3. Create a walking group in your office to walk around your neighborhood after lunch.

4. If you are at home during lunch, walk around your block or hop on a treadmill after you eat.

5. If the weather doesn't permit you to get outside, walk around inside your office for a few minutes after you eat. Take the stairs up a few floors, or stroll over to another department to visit a colleague. Even a little movement after you eat will have a beneficial effect on your energy level.

20

Make Tonight Your Night

You have had a long day. All you feel like doing when you get home is crashing on the couch. After all, this is what you usually do. But then someone like me comes along and says it doesn't have to be this way. I ask you if you would like to have more energy in the evening. You say, "Yes." I ask you if you would rather be active than sitting on a couch in the evening. You say, "Yes . . . if only I had the energy I would be more active." Try these simple changes to your evening routine that can make all the difference.

> "The difference between one man and another is not mere ability it is energy."
> —THOMAS ARNOLD

ACTION STEPS

1. Eat an energizing snack before dinner. According to William Nagler, M.D., psychiatrist at the University of California, Los Angeles School of Medicine, evidence indicates simple hunger-related tensions contribute to fading energy, negative emotions, and late-day arguments. When you eat a snack before dinner you will most likely be in better spirits and eat less for dinner.

2. Create a buffer zone. Take 15–20 minutes to be by yourself after walking in the door before having conversations about personal, financial, or professional matters. According to Dr. Cooper, evidence suggests over half of the most damaging arguments are started or magnified within 15 minutes of people greeting each other at the end of the day. Now I know why my mother said, "Don't talk to your father until he has eaten dinner." When we take the time to walk in the house, get comfortable, and then engage in conversations and family time, we will likely have less stressful conversations.

3. Eat smaller dinners. Eat enough to satisfy you, but not so much that you want to go to bed after eating.

4. Take a light 10-minute walk after dinner. Instead of plopping down to watch TV take a walk. Walking after dinner, within a half-hour time frame is like pouring gasoline on a fire. It exponentially increases your metabolism and gives you a double boost of energy according to Bryant Stamford, Ph.D., exercise physiologist at the University of Louisville. You will also likely eat less high fat foods and be in a better mood.

5. Play at night. Do some effortless gardening, or play with your kids or pet. Playing at night helps us combat fatigue and stress.

6. Reflect. Think about all the things you are thankful for and say "thank you." I like to go outside and look at the stars (a benefit of living at the beach is that you can see them) and think about how lucky I am to be alive.

21

Notice the Effects of Exercise

There is a lot of well-documented evidence that supports the claim exercise reduces stress, increases energy and makes people healthier. However, we don't really need anyone to tell us working out is good for us—we know it firsthand from our own experiences and feelings. When we take a jog and break a sweat, we feel good. When we take a long walk and get our blood pumping through our bodies we feel energized. We may feel a little sore the next day if we haven't exercised in a while, but the soreness quickly subsides and is replaced by strength and power.

If you're like me, exercise helps you put all of the little annoying life problems, that otherwise would consume you, into perspective. For instance, my wife is always worried about paying the bills, calling the gas company, getting our daughter new clothes for school, finding a babysitter for Saturday night, and a thousand other nuisances. However, when she goes to the gym, she returns worry-free, with a feeling that everything will work out just fine. When she feels this way, strangely enough, it always does.

"If exercise could be packaged into a pill, it would be the single most prescribed and beneficial medicine in the nation."
—ROBERT BUTLER, M.D., MOUNT SINAI MEDICAL CENTER

Exercise helps us build muscle and reduce fat, but it also clears our minds, strengthens our heart, reduces our stress, and energizes our lives.

Research shows that exercise is as equally effective as antidepressants for mild and moderate depression. After an exercise session, we have a positive outlook on the world and believe that we can take on anything.

ACTION STEPS

1. **Notice how you feel after you've exercised. Think about the physical effects exercise has on your body, but also the effects it has on your emotions. Write these sensations down.**

2. **The next time you start to consider skipping your workout, look at your writing and remember how good exercise makes you feel, physically and emotionally.**

22

Straighten Up

Did you know that poor posture can reduce the amount of oxygen you take in to your lungs by more than 30 percent? This means less oxygen for your body and brain . . . and less energy for you.

Much of the research also suggests poor posture affects more than just your oxygen intake. It also influences the way you feel, think, and act. According to Rene Cailliet, M.D., chairman of the department of physical medicine at the Santa Monica Hospital Center, when you're stooped over, you not only look old and out of touch with life, but you also tend to *feel* that way.

"Stand up straight!"
—MOM

In a technology driven world, maintaining good posture is no easy task. Many of our jobs require us to sit at a desk looking at a computer screen all day. We have become afflicted with a 21st-century disease I call Head Forwarditis—leaning forward with our head and following with our shoulders. With each forward slouch we're cutting the supply of oxygen to our lungs, decreasing our energy and affecting our attitude.

But there is a solution. If we pay attention to our posture and focus on standing and sitting up straight, we can make significant changes in how we feel and think. Experts know (and we know from our experiences and observations) that the link between our posture and attitude is bi-directional. Posture can affect your attitude, just as attitude affects your posture. I consider this great news—science is telling us that we have one more tool to improve our attitude and increase our energy. Posture expert Wilfred Barlow, M.D., says, "We're not born knowing how to do it right—we have to learn it." No matter our height, we can practice sitting tall, walking tall and thinking tall. We can "straighten up" for increased energy.

ACTION STEPS

1. Practice standing and sitting up straight as much as possible. Imagine an invisible force gently tugging at the top of your head—lifting your head, lengthening your neck, pulling your shoulders back and down, and straightening your back.

2. Make it a habit to focus on your posture every 30 minutes. Eventually great posture will feel natural.

3. When you are feeling sad or upset, pay even more attention to your posture. Force yourself to "straighten up."

23

Tone Your Tummy

Your abdominal muscles are a key source of strength and energy. Strong abdominal muscles help you maintain better posture which helps you breathe better and inhale more energizing oxygen into your lungs. This means more energy for your brain and body. While stomach exercises are most everyone's least favorite exercise, they are essential to a strong abdominal region and increased energy.

I have found the stomach crunch to be the most effective ab exercise. Stomach crunches, when done properly, allow you to focus on building your stomach muscles without hurting your back. Stomach exercises should include slow and steady movements in order to maximize the tension placed on the stomach muscles. Avoid fast, uncontrolled movements that may cause you harm. As with any exercise, I recommend you consult an exercise book such as *Body for Life*, a magazine such as *Shape,* a physical trainer, or a physician. One session with a physical trainer should be enough to teach you the basics. Here are a few tips to help you tone your tummy.

ACTION STEPS

1. Do your stomach exercises in the morning when you get out of bed. All it takes is a few minutes each morning to increase your energy for a lifetime. At first this habit will take getting used to but soon it will become a natural part of your routine.

2. If the morning isn't a good time for your abdominal exercises, then change into comfortable clothes and do your exercises when you get home from work—before TV, dinner, or any other evening activity.

24

Smell a Little Energy

Has the smell of the autumn air ever reminded you of a specific fall day in your past? Or have you ever noticed someone's perfume or cologne and been swept into the memory of a past relationship? If so, you have already experienced the power of smell in your life. In fact, our sense of smell is so powerfully connected to the brain that some scents elicit pronounced changes in energy, emotions, and memory. In fact, there is growing evidence that the power of smell can, at least in some cases, strongly influence mental alertness.

> **"Smell is a potent wizard that transports us across thousands of miles and all the years we have lived."**
> **—HELEN KELLER**

Study after study demonstrates the power of smell. At Rensselaer Polytechnic Institute, researchers showed people who work in pleasantly scented areas performed 25 percent better than those in unscented areas. The people in pleasantly scented rooms carried out their tasks more confidently and more efficiently. Tests at the University of Cincinnati indicate fragrances added to the atmosphere of a room can help keep people more alert and improve performance of routine tasks.

So what smells energize us? Peppermint and lemon seem to be most effective, but scent is a deeply personal sense. Experiment to see which one, if either, is the right one for you. The smell of rosemary is also reportedly effective for uplifting energy and enhancing memory. However, rosemary shouldn't be used by women who are pregnant or anyone with high blood pressure. Try these steps to use scent to energize your life.

ACTION STEPS

1. At different times, try a cup of peppermint tea and lemon tea. Take in the strong fragrant vapors and see which one has the stronger effect. Drink the tea that energizes you the most.

2. Open a bottle of peppermint extract and lemon extract (available at most health food stores). Whichever pleases your senses the most is the right one for you.

3. Once you decide which smell energizes you the most, consider using a scent dispenser to dispense all-natural essential oils wherever you work or live.

4. Bring fresh flowers or potpourri into your home or work areas.

25

Find the Light

Have you ever stood outside for a few minutes and felt your body soaking in the sun like a solar panel fueling up with energy?

Well, scientists now tell us there is a link between exposure to light and our energy levels. In a three-year study conducted at Harvard University, Drs. Richard Kronauer and Charles Czeisler were able to link the impact of light on the retina of the eye to better attention focus and energy production in the brain. Other studies have shown that the body has hundreds of biochemical and hormonal rhythms, all keyed to light and dark, and that the human brain is powerfully affected when the body is exposed to bright light.

Doctors also know that seasonal affective disorder, also called "the winter blues," can be treated with exposure to sunlight or full spectrum lighting produced by light machines that mimic sunlight. Exposure to sunlight also enhances our immune system and facilitates our skin's production of Vitamin D—leading to healthier teeth and bones.

While the benefits of finding the light are clear, please remember to make your time in the sun brief. We not only receive the greatest benefits from brief sunlight exposure, but we also know the health consequences associated with spending too much time in the sun can be dire.

ACTION STEPS

1. Exercise in the morning and soak up some morning sunlight.
2. Take a brief "sun break" during your lunch break.
3. Use sunscreen daily, and always reapply when you'll be exposed to direct sunlight for longer periods of time.

26

Breathe in Energy and Breathe out Worries

One of the most simple and powerful ways to increase your energy is to breathe. That's right. Breathe. We all do it, but sometimes we forget to do it right. When we get stressed, research tells us, we take shorter breaths and get less oxygen into our lungs. This means less oxygen in the brain and body and less energy for you.

Each time you feel yourself getting stressed, focus on your breathing. Take in five to ten deep breaths. Rather than shallow breaths, focus on energizing breaths. Breathe in energy and breathe out today's worries. So as you live, work, shop, clean, run errands, do the laundry, get together with friends, make time for family and attack your to-do list, monitor yourself and ask *Am I stressed? Am I breathing?*

ACTION STEPS

Practice your energizer breath now.

1. **Get comfortable. Loosen your shoulders and neck.**
2. **Exhale completely.**

3. Inhale through your nose for a silent count of three.
4. Hold your breath for a few seconds.
5. Exhale through your mouth for a silent count of four (focus on your breathing).
6. Repeat five to ten times (imagine each breath fueling you up with breathing).

27

Don't Swim Against the Current

Human beings, like all things in nature, experience cycles. The earth rotates, causing day and night. The tides go in, the tides go out. The seasons change, and our energy rises and falls many times within a twenty-four-hour cycle.

In order to maximize your energy it is important to pay attention to your energy and notice when it is rising and falling. Do you feel a wave of energy coming on? Or is your energy meter at zero and everything you do is a struggle? Is the energy flowing or is it fighting? These observations help you use your energy cycles to your advantage. When you feel a surge of energy you can then ride the wave. Like a great surfer you can take that wave higher and farther, performing incredible feats along the way. Salespeople make their most effective sales calls during this time. A stay-at-home parent can do the housework of five people. A writer can write twice as much in the same amount of time.

"When we take time to catch our breath and look around, a heartbeat can be found in the earth's deep constant rhythms."
—ALEXANDRA CIPUZAK

In contrast, when your energy is at a low point you don't want to fight against the current. Instead of asking yourself *Why am I so tired right now?* and drinking coffee or an artificial energy booster to fight your downturns, there is another way. During moments of low energy, don't fight the current. Take a short energy break. Go outside and get some fresh air. Drink a bottle of water. Five to ten minutes will make the difference. This will help you recharge instead of draining more energy. Then when your energy surges again you can take full advantage.

When you ride your waves and flow with the current you will most likely notice what I noticed: that you are more productive and do not get burned out. Someone who constantly fights against the current with fake energy boosters may succeed in the short run but in the end their mind and body will wear down. Depriving yourself of sleep, breaks, and your body's biological needs will eventually take its toll. At some point sales will decline. Housework will be left undone and writer's block will set in. In contrast a person who learns to flow with their energy will have more energy when they need it.

ACTION STEPS

1. **Pay attention to your energy levels throughout the day.**
2. **When you feel a surge of energy, ride the wave.**
3. **When you feel like your energy is crashing, take a short break.**

28

Take Short Energy Breaks

Just as athletes need to take water breaks, we need to take short energy breaks to survive and thrive. In today's fast-paced, 24/7, don't-stop-till-you-drop culture, we too often push our minds and bodies to the max without regard for rest or sleep. Family life and career life ask more and more of us, requiring us to ask more and more of ourselves. We often tell ourselves we'll take a break when we're done with the latest house project or the newest business deal. We say we'll relax when the holidays are here or when school is out. The problem is, it's not getting any easier—the demands on our time will continue to grow, and our energy will continue to decrease if we don't change. We can't change society, so we have to change ourselves.

The key is to take short energy breaks during our busy day. Even a one-minute break can help us find the calm in the midst of chaos. Dr. Etienne Grandjean, a productivity expert at the Swiss Polytechnic Institute, has studied human performance, and he suggests that people who take short breaks have a greater number of total accomplishments per day and exhibit less distress and fatigue. As a general rule, try to take a short break at least every few hours.

> **"The best know how to rest."**
> **—ALAN COHEN**

ACTION STEPS

1. If you work in an office, stand up and stretch at your desk, or go outside and stretch and loosen up your shoulders.
2. If you are home, take a walk around the block.
3. Shift your gaze. Give your eyes a break by looking at something else. If you stare at a computer screen all day, look away. Look at the window. Stand up and look across the room.
4. Find a rest room sink and splash cold water on your face.
5. Eat a healthy snack.
6. Sip ice water. With each sip you increase your energy and alertness.
7. Close your eyes and focus on your breathing for five minutes.
8. Visit with a colleague or neighbor and share a story or a joke.
9. Call your significant other for a quick chat.

29

Energize with Yoga

The word "yoga" is a Sanskrit term that means "union" or "joining." Teachers explain yoga is the joining or uniting of the mind, body and spirit to improve our life, and enhance our health.

Hatha yoga is the branch of yoga that is based on physical postures called *asanas*—of which there are thousands—and breath controls, called *pranayama*. Hatha yoga helps a person connect with inner energy, quiets a busy mind, and increases physical, mental and spiritual energy. The physical and mental aspects of yoga help your mind and body become one. The spiritual aspects help you become one with the energy of everything. With each pose and breath you connect with your own energy and the energy of the universe. Yoga helps you increase your flexibility and tones your muscles. I used to have neck problems and pinched nerves until I started yoga and now I am pain-free.

> **"What lies before us and what lies behind us is nothing compared to what lies within us."**
> **—RALPH WALDO EMERSON**

Yoga also includes breathing exercises that help you focus your mind and body on the present moment. With each breath you fill your body with energy and unite the energy outside you with the energy inside you. With yoga, everything is right here, right now. With each breath, each movement, and each moment of silence you unite and energize your mind, body, and spirit.

And one of the best things about yoga is that you don't need equipment or a special room. All you need is you and a small area of space. With yoga you can energize your life anytime, anywhere.

ACTION STEPS

1. Visit *Yoga Journal* (www.yogajournal.com) for postures, techniques, and information. Other sources of information: www.yoga.com for articles and books and www.yrec.org for the philosophical underpinnings of yoga.

2. Check out a yoga video for a few weeks from your library or local video store.

3. Introduce your kids to yoga. The natural animal-like poses are very easy for kids to follow. My three-year-old son loves doing the cobra and cat poses.

4. Forget Twister. It's time for Yoga. A new trend is taking place where instructors will come to your home and teach yoga poses at a party. This also works especially well for kids' parties.

5. My favorite yoga teacher, speaker, and trainer is Megan McDonough. Visit her at www.urinfinityinabox.com. As a business yogi she helps people work with ease using introspective yoga techniques.

30

Connect with Nature

Ever wonder why people love the beach, the mountains, and places like Central Park in New York City? Because they are powerful sources of energy. Whether it's the ocean air, the crashing waves, large trees or fields of green, when we visit these places we feel the positive energy of nature, and it has a profound effect on our mind and body.

My friend Deb says that she gets her energy from the beach. She once told me, "The sunlight reflecting off the water gives me energy and the waves crashing on shore give me strength."

I have a friend, Brian, who loves to hike in the mountains. He says that he goes to the mountains to put his life in perspective. And many of the residents of New York City will tell you Central Park is where they recharge their batteries.

> **"All beings are encompassed within one all-encompassing great energy: So I understood from the coolness of this morning's passing breeze."**
> **—MUMON**

If you are like most people, you probably are reading this thinking: *Yes, I love these places. I feel great when I go there.* And like most people it's probably been so long since you have tapped the energy of nature that you forgot how much you loved going to these places until you read this. Well, I urge you now to remember the feeling you get when you sit in the park, or feel hot sand on your feet, or stand under 100-year-old trees and let this feeling motivate you to take the time to connect with nature and enjoy the energy it will generously share with you.

ACTION STEPS

1. Visit a place of nature at least once a week. Pick a time and a day and make it a ritual. Take your lunch break in a nearby park.
2. Ride your bike to the beach. Take your kids hiking in the mountains. Go fishing at a nearby lake. Exercise with a friend in a park.
3. If you love golf, consider a visit to the golf course as beneficial as a trip to the park so long as you take the time to enjoy the air, the trees and the green grass.
4. Connect with nature and connect often.

31

Add the Energy of Play to Your Day

Did you know that children laugh about 400 times a day, while adults laugh only about 25 times? If you need more energy for your life and career, then add a little play to your day. When you play, your life flows easier and your day flows faster.

If you feel you've forgotten how to play, simply watch children. They always seem to have boundless energy, perhaps because they're always laughing and playing. They are full of life, energy, and smiles. Without a thought for tomorrow they truly enjoy the present.

> **"If you wish to glimpse inside a human soul, just watch a person laugh and play. Those who laugh and play well are the most alive."**
> —FYODOR DOSTOYEVSKY

I have two children, and having fun and not being stressed about them has been one of the big challenges in my life. While they played I would worry about them getting hurt or dirty. But through this challenge I have learned that if I behave more like them and less like a stressed-out adult, I will be happier—and so will my family. When it comes to play, my children are my teachers.

ACTION STEPS

1. Tell a joke. Make someone laugh today, and you'll find yourself laughing as well. In California, the new rage is laughing clubs where people get together and simply laugh.

2. Smile. The simple act of smiling can improve your mood and increase your energy.

3. Play with your kids. Roll around the grass with them. Play tag. Eat ice cream together.

4. Dance the night away. Sometimes when I'm writing during the day or night, my wife will put on music downstairs. I'll walk down from my office and she and the kids will be jumping around and dancing. At first they look funny, but once I start dancing with them I feel energized and rejuvenated. (Plus, the visual of my little kids dancing just makes me laugh.)

5. Get back to your favorite hobby. Remember that thing that you used to love doing? Make time once a day—or at least once a week—to do it.

6. Play at work. My friend Teddy works on Wall Street. Teddy is famous for having fun and playing games. Even at work Teddy finds a way to play. His personal game: he tries to answer the phone quicker than anyone in his company. While this may be silly to some, Teddy says it makes him sharper and his day flow faster. What can you do to make work more fun?

Play after work. My friend Amy is a pharmaceutical rep by day and comedian by night. Doing what she loves after work makes her more fulfilled and productive during the day.

32

Recharge Your Batteries with the Energy of Sleep

> "Failure is more frequently from want of energy than want of capital."
>
> —DANIEL WEBSTER

I have heard many people say sleep is overrated. That is, until they don't get enough of it.

While there are a few people who can consistently get by with only four hours of sleep per night, most of us require at least eight hours of sleep—and nine to ten hours a night is optimal, according to Cornell Psychology Professor James B. Maas. One-third of Americans get less than six hours of sleep a night. Research shows that if you get less than eight hours of sleep, you are operating in an "impaired" state; your alertness, productivity, creativity, and general health are all affected. We all know about the risks of driving while impaired . . . but living in a perpetually impaired state is another matter altogether.

According to Mass, "Between the seventh and eighth hour of sleep is when we get almost an hour of REM (rapid eye movement) sleep, the time when the mind repairs itself, grows new connections and recharges us. If you only sleep six hours a night, you're missing that last, important opportunity to repair and to prepare for the coming day." This means less energy for your body and less energy for you.

Who wants to live life impaired like this? And why should we have to? Instead of only sleeping six to seven hours a night and operating on half a battery, we can sleep eight to ten hours a night and charge our battery to the max. Here are a few action steps to help you get eight to ten hours of sleep a night.

ACTION STEPS

1. Decide what time you need to go to bed to get at least eight hours of sleep a night.

2. In your daily planner write down that time and make sure you are in bed ten minutes before that time. Note the first few nights may be difficult to fall asleep. Keep in mind you are training yourself and your body.

3. To help you go to sleep, avoid sugars and caffeine before bed. Eat a snack if you are hungry. Exercise during the day, but not right before bed.

4. Clear your mind and say to yourself, "It's time to go to bed. I deserve to sleep." If your mind starts whirling, use this self-talk to help you tune out your thoughts. Tell yourself, "I can think all about this tomorrow. Now is the time for me to sleep."

5. Go to bed each night at the same time. Eventually you will get used to going to bed at that time.

6 **Observe your energy in the morning and throughout the day as you get more sleep each night.**

7 **For more information on sleeping well visit www.sleepfoundation.org.**

33

Take a Power Nap

My grandfather Eddy told me that one of the keys to his long and energetic life is a daily short power nap. At eighty-five years of age he still takes one. While not everyone may need a daily power nap, for those who are not getting enough sleep at night, a power nap will help you refresh your mind and body during the day. Cornell psychologist Dr. James Maas, author of *Power Sleep*, says a twenty-minute nap in the afternoon actually provides more rest than sleeping an extra twenty minutes in the morning. According to Charles McPhee, also known as the "Dream Doctor," naps should be performed at midday—about eight hours after we wake up—so as to not disturb the natural biorhythm of our sleep-wake cycles. He also says, "Naps also should be short, definitely no longer than thirty minutes. (Longer naps allow us to settle into deep sleep, from which it is difficult to awaken)."

While sleep experts are recommending corporations provide nap rooms for their employees to increase their productivity, many bosses still do not understand the benefits of a power nap. So what's an Energy Addict who works in an office to do to recharge their midday battery?

ACTION STEPS

1. While others are taking their 20-minute coffee break, take a 20-minute power nap.

2. The Dream Doctor says not to worry if you don't fall asleep. Just closing your eyes and relaxing peacefully will be refreshing.

3. To prevent yourself from napping too long, the Dream Doctor recommends you set an alarm for 15–30 minutes on your watch or cell phone. This will also help you rest more peacefully.

4. If all else fails, the Dream Doctor recommends the ten best things to say if you get caught napping at your desk at www.dreamdoctor.com. My two favorites:

   - "This is just a 15-minute power-nap like they raved about in that time-management course you sent me to."
   - "I wasn't sleeping! I was meditating on our mission statement."

34

Make Technology Work for You

Computers, mobile phones, wireless web phones, pagers, PDAs and every other new gadget made with the latest technology is supposed to make our lives better. The marketers promote every new innovation as the product that will transform our lives, give us more time, make us more productive, and provide us with the freedom and power to go wherever and do whatever we want. In many ways, they are right. The potentials of new technologies are as great as the claims. However, in reality, the use (or misuse) of technology falls considerably short of the promises.

We see people talking on the mobile phone in a restaurant, instead of talking to the person across the table. We hear a person's entire conversation on the train as he talks into his earpiece. We feel tethered to our desks, compelled to check our e-mail constantly throughout the day. On average, about five pagers and phones go off in the movie theater during the course of a two-hour movie. Communication devices that should give us more freedom actually become tracking devices so that anyone can find us anytime, anywhere. In reality technology makes life more complicated rather than making it easier.

Don't blame technology. It's our fault—we allow technology

to rule our lives instead of making technology work for us. We need to stop being a slave to our phone and computer and other gadgets and become a master of our technology-filled world.

This doesn't mean we need to get rid of technology. Rather we need to make technology work for us.

ACTION STEPS

1. Shut off your phone. It's as easy as pressing the power button when you don't want to be disturbed.

2. Ignore the call-waiting feature. Focus on the person you are talking to and you'll feel better too.

3. Check your e-mail only three times a day. This will help you be more productive and focus on what you have to do instead of checking every five minutes to see if someone e-mailed you.

35

Use the Magical "Off" Button

This simple strategy has helped me escape from my cell—cell phone, that is. Where I once was confined, I now am free because I found the "off" button that liberated me. Think about it.

When your phone is always ringing and you're doing three things at once, your energy is being scattered in many different directions. You can't help but feel uneasy and stressed out. Your energy doesn't want to be in three different places at once. It wants to be in one place. Shutting off your phone allows you to focus your energy now, on the people you are talking to now, and on the matters that need your attention in front of you now. When you are finished dealing with these situations, you can turn your phone back on to handle other situations.

When you first start shutting your phone off, you will experience a little separation anxiety—but soon that will be replaced by a new feeling of power. The phone is not a prison. It is a tool for you to communicate when you need to use it. It is meant to make you more successful, not scattered and tired. So don't let your cell phone drain your energy. Shut it off until you are ready to use it.

ACTION STEP

There is nothing in the user's manual that says your phone or pager must stay on 24/7. If you don't want to be bothered during a movie, dinner, at home, or during a conversation, just shut the phone off and let your voicemail accept the call. When you are ready to talk, simply turn your phone on, check your messages, and call people back on your time instead of theirs. You'll be amazed at how simply shutting off your phone at certain times will help you focus and increase your energy.

36

Ignore the Call-Waiting Feature

How many times have we been on a call and we hear the dreaded "beep"? I don't know about you, it makes me feel unimportant when the person that I'm talking to checks to see who else is calling. It also takes a lot of energy to maintain several conversations at once. "Clickers" waste a lot of energy going back and forth from one conversation to another, in many cases for several hours a day. Half the time they can't even remember to whom they are speaking. I have been in the presence of many clickers and they always appear frantic, disorganized and chaotic.

Shouldn't we just reserve the call-waiting feature for times when we are waiting for the doctor to call or the real estate agent to say that our house has been sold? Shouldn't we give the person on the other line the attention they deserve? And shouldn't we do it most of all for ourselves and our own energy's sake? Most phone systems have voice mail that will answer when you are on the other line. When you are done speaking, you can check your messages and call people back. When you ignore the call-waiting feature, you will notice your conversations are more meaningful and you don't feel as scattered. You can focus on one conversation and exchange positive calm energy with the person on the other end of the phone, rather than hurrying from one caller to the next.

ACTION STEP

Try ignoring call-waiting for a week and observe how your experience of talking on the phone changes. Hear the difference in your conversations, and feel how your focused conversations with one person at a time actually feeds you with energy.

37

Eliminate Clutter: Inside and Out

Do you have a new project that needs to get done? Perhaps a proposal you should prepare for a new client, or the first chapter of the book you have always wanted to write. Maybe it's a song that has been floating in your head or a plan for your new business. If there is something that you need to do but it's not getting done, one of the first places to start is to clear out the clutter around you and inside you.

Clutter can block precious new energy from flowing into your life by filling up your space and life with old stagnant energy—energy that loves to build up and stay right where it is. Clutter in your life might include a messy house, a pile of papers on your desk, mail spread out all over the counter, a closet filled with old clothes you never wear, or even those old salad dressings taking up space in your refrigerator.

When you attack that to-do list, you clear the physical energy around you and allow new energy to flow in. It's an energy thing. It simply makes you feel better. We are energy, so when we clear out the old stagnant energy around our space we feel more lively and energized.

The same goes for mental clutter. When you get rid of toxic thoughts, toxic people and toxic beliefs in your life you eliminate the energetic clutter that holds you back. Replace beliefs such as

"Bad things always happen to me" with "I accept all the great things in my life." Replace thoughts like "I hate the rain" to "I love the rain because it brings us water and life." This is one I have worked on a lot. And to the people who are always being negative to you and filling your life with negative words and actions, ask them to change. Try to help them change. If they are unwilling, you just might have to throw them and their clutter out of your life.

Once you clear your clutter, you'll feel more energized and alive. You'll have new energy to start your project and create new success in your life. Try it and you'll feel the difference.

ACTION STEPS

1. **Pick one space in your house and/or office that is cluttered. Organize it and throw out the clutter. Observe how you feel when you are finished.**
2. **Identify one toxic person, thought, or belief in your life and change it. Feel how your energy increases.**
3. **Keep a journal to help release clutter from your mind.**
4. **Read the books *Clear Your Clutter with Feng Shui* by Karen Kingston and *Organizing from the Inside Out* by Julie Morganstern.**

38

Find Your Song and Play the Music

Most of us have a favorite song that lifts us up whenever we hear it. You're sitting in your car and your favorite song will come on the radio. You start singing along, and before you know it your day has turned around from frustration to joy. Music is energy that vibrates—just as the approximately 75 trillion cells in our body vibrate. When we hear music, our bodies will often feel the music before we even realize we are moving to the beat.

> **"Drumsound rises on the air, its throb, my heart. A voice inside the beat says, 'I know you're tired, but come. This is the way.' "**
>
> —RUMI

Music has the power to make us laugh and cry. Think of the music from the movies *Terms of Endearment* and *Titanic.* The music starts playing and the audience is reaching for tissues. Music also has the power to motivate us and inspire us. Think of the *Rocky* movies. When I hear the theme song I still get the urge to sprint a hundred yards.

Music sets the tone in restaurants and shopping malls. It plays during sporting events, religious services, and family holidays. After all, what would a birthday be without a rousing chorus of the *Happy Birthday* song?

Music makes us think and feel because it is a powerful source of energy and each day you have the opportunity to make the energy of music work for you. When you are down you can play a song that lifts your spirit and adds a kick to your step. When you are going to an important meeting or event, you can play a song that gives you confidence. When you are stressed and nervous you can play music that relaxes you. Music is energy that you can use to fuel your life whenever and wherever you need it.

ACTION STEP

Technology makes it easier than ever to energize your life with music. Most music stores now have machines that allow you to make custom CDs. Or you can use a computer to store your favorite CDs and with your computer and a CD burner you can make your own energizing CD. Make a list of the songs that lift you up and create your custom CD or tape. When you feel down or need a pick-me-up, find your song and play the music.

39

Create Your Energy Addict Kit

I own a small black gym bag that I now call my Energy Addict Kit. Inside this bag, I keep many of my power sources. A box of raisins, a bag of nuts, and a container of trail mix are a few of the healthy snacks I carry with me. My kit also contains a bottle of vitamins, sneakers for walking, two of my favorite books, my favorite movie, my favorite songs on a CD, a box of green tea, a bottle of Penta Water, and a picture of my wife and kids. I consider the contents of this bag fuel for my life. When I am feeling hungry and tired, my snack is within reach. If I forgot to take my vitamins in the morning, they are available in my bag. If I feel sluggish after lunch, a light walk with my sneakers usually does the trick. I never get fatigued from lack of water with my bottle near me, and I can always energize my mind with a great book, a cup of green tea, an uplifting song, an inspiring movie, or simply a meaningful picture of my wife and kids. My kit is truly a bag full of energy.

I encourage you to create your own Energy Addict Kit. As an Energy Addict you'll always want the positive, powerful sources of energy you are addicted to within reach. The great thing about an Energy Addict Kit is we can all create our own customized contents. By reading this book and discovering the power sources in your life, you can start to build your own kit and incorporate your power sources into your daily routine. Think of it this way—doctors need specific instruments to be helpful. Plumbers need their tool kit to be effective. Artists need their paint and paper to create. And Energy Addicts need great sources of energy to thrive. An Energy Addict Kit helps you bring many of your power sources into one mobile, accessible bag that is available whenever and wherever you need some fuel.

ACTION STEPS

1. Convert a gym bag or bag of your choice into your Energy Addict Kit.
2. Decide what power sources you would like to add to your kit.
3. Bring your kit to your office or on the road when you are driving or traveling.
4. Whenever you need some fuel, reach into your kit and do what Energy Addicts do best—use great sources of energy to create success in their lives.

PART 2

MENTAL STRATEGIES

40

Start Your Day Off Right

A new client of mine called me up the other day and said, "I always crash in the afternoon. What can I do?"

I said to him, "I bet I can guess your morning routine. You hit the snooze button a few times. Jump out of bed. Rush to the shower. Gulp a cup of coffee and rush out the door. You yell at a few people for driving slowly on the road. Get to your desk. You have e-mails in your in-box and voicemails you haven't returned. The day starts and you're tired already."

"That's me," he said. "How did you know?"

He's not alone. But when we spend our morning rushing around, our bodies run on stress hormones instead of "real energy." Stress hormones send flight-or-fight responses through your system, causing you to have more energy temporarily. Like a person in a fight, energy increases dramatically. However, if you have ever been in a fight, you know afterward your energy is drained and you feel exhausted. Your stress hormones will give you energy now, but cause you to crash later.

> **"When you arise in the morning, think of what a precious privilege it is to be alive—to breathe, to think, to enjoy, to love."**
> **—MARCUS AURELIUS**

The key to increased energy is to start your day off right and fuel your morning with your sustained power sources instead of stress hormones. Earlier in this book, we talked about some important physical aspects to starting your morning—eating breakfast and exercising. But there are some other actions you can take to start off the day in a positive and energized frame of mind.

ACTION STEPS

1. Awake to music instead of a beeping alarm. Researchers say this helps you awake more peacefully instead of shocking your body and brain out of sleep. Keep the volume high enough to wake you but not so high that it startles you.

2. Don't hit the snooze button. Give yourself enough time to engage in an energizing morning instead of having to rush around.

3. Find the light. Many studies report that when we expose our body and brain to bright light we increase our alertness and energy. Turn on a lamp, go to a window, or walk outside—the light helps you get ready to take on the day.

4. Think positive thoughts. Instead of being fearful and anxious, causing a release of stress hormones, thinking positively about the day will send positive energy to your body supplying you with sustained energy.

5. Get inspired. Instead of reading the latest news of violence and scandals, read something that energizes you. Perhaps a quote book, or *Simple Abundance,* or the *Bible*.

41

Neutralize the Energy Vampires

They lurk in our businesses, our families, and our social organizations. They are real. They are everywhere. And they will suck the life out of you if you let them. They're the Energy Vampires.

> **"I will not let anyone walk through my mind with their dirty feet."**
> **—MAHATMA GANDHI**

If you're like most people, it has happened to you. You start talking to someone and, before you know it, they've drained the energy and excitement right out of you. You look for fang marks on your neck, but then you realize Energy Vampires don't have fangs—they have other means to suck your energy.

- **Negative comments.** "Did I tell you how much I hate my life and work? Did I tell you what so and so did to me? Did I tell you how my life stinks? Did I tell you why nothing goes right?"
- **Dream snatching.** "You can't do that. How are you going to do that? Are you living in fantasyland? Get back to the real world. You should do this instead."
- **Shrinking devices.** "What is wrong with you? Can you do anything right? You are the worst. I hate working with you."

In other situations the words may be less harsh, but the result ends up being the same. Once an Energy Vampire starts sucking it is difficult to break free. Don't let this happen. Instead be prepared to neutralize an Energy Vampire from the beginning. You don't need a stake or garlic.

ACTION STEPS

1. Look in the mirror. Sometimes we are the Vampires. If we pay attention to our thoughts and words we can eliminate the vampire in us. Are you being negative or positive?

2. Confront and reform. Tell your Energy Vampire (EV) that he or she is being negative. They may not even realize it. Ask for support, positive feedback, and encouragement from them. If your EV is a colleague, family member, or friend, perhaps you can reform them into an Energy Addict. Show them how to spread positive energy.

3. Turn on the light. When you were a child and scared of the dark you turned on the light and felt better. Negative energy is like darkness. When you encounter an Energy Vampire, turn on the light. When an EV comes at you with fear, negativity, hate, and anger, respond with love, kindness, and positive energy. Negative energy is powerless in the light.

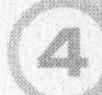

Run. Run as far and as fast as you can. Really fast. This sometimes is the best technique if you are not close with the EV. You only have so much energy, and in today's world you need to keep all you have.

Identify one EV in your life and decide what technique you will use to neutralize them.

42

Transform Energy into Results

What turns an idea into a reality? A vision into a painting? Words into a poem? Like everything in nature, we possess the enormous power to focus energy in order to create. The miraculous power of a woman's body to channel and focus the necessary energy to create and birth a baby is one of nature's greatest gifts. While not everyone has the ability to create human life, we all have the power to give life to our ideas, plans, and dreams. We can birth a painting, a building, an invention. Everything we create is a result of our focused energy.

In one state, energy is passive—sitting and waiting to be used. A pen sitting on a table. A plan not yet read. A road not yet taken. In another state, energy is scattered—a fire out of control, a person being pulled in a thousand different directions. In the desired state, energy is focused. The words written, a plan acted upon, a person in pursuit of his or her goals.

> **"Most people have no idea of the giant capacity we can immediately command when we focus all of our resources on mastering a single area of our lives."**
> **—ANTHONY ROBBINS**

We have the opportunity every day to channel our scattered energy into focused energy. We can grab the energy being scattered and wasted on things we don't really want and focus that energy on creating the life we do want. Just as an architect designs a building, we have the ability to design our life. The design determines what we build, the tools and materials needed and the energy required. Just as a builder applies his or her energy to transform the design into reality, we must grab a set of tools, focus our actions, thoughts and words and create our life—one positive thought, one action at a time.

ACTION STEPS

1. Write down what you want to create. These are your goals. The act of writing your goals begins the process of transforming your thoughts into your reality. For instance, one of your goals might be to increase your energy.

2. Decide what steps are necessary to achieve your goals. If your goal is to increase your energy you might write:

   Eat breakfast.
   Exercise in the morning.
   Have more fun.

3. Create a schedule and/or plan to incorporate your action steps into your life. For this example you might write:

   Eat breakfast before work Monday-Friday. Eat breakfast by 7 am.
   Do 5–10 minutes of exercise Monday-Thursday at 6:30 am.
   Play a game with the kids after dinner Monday and Wednesday.

4. Add this schedule to your calendar or planner. It needs to be as important as a meeting with your doctor.

43

Zoom Focus on the Little Things

In addition to focusing your energy to achieve your goals there is another kind of focus you will need. While focusing on your yearly and weekly goals requires a big-picture focus, there is something I call Zoom Focus. Zoom Focus is all about focusing day-to-day and minute-to-minute.

In today's hurried technology-driven society, Zoom Focus is more important than ever. Each day the difference between success and failure is found in the little things. Little phone calls can waste precious time. Little disruptions can disturb critical moments of concentration. And little interruptions that come in many forms can waste your most valuable asset—your energy. Zoom Focus means we focus on doing the right little things that lead to success and stop letting the wrong little things waste our time and energy.

Implementing Zoom Focus involves several of the same action steps as we discussed for the Large Goals. However, the results can be seen much sooner—instant gratification!

ACTION STEPS

1. Carry a small notebook or planner with you.

2. In the morning before you go to work or right when you get to work, write down your priorities for the day. What are the little things you need to focus on today? Today it may be paperwork.

3. Then write down the little roadblocks that can get in the way. What has become a roadblock in the past, and what do you anticipate blocking your focus today? For example, if you planned on getting a lot of paperwork done today, one of the roadblocks might be phone calls and e-mails from friends and family.

4. Decide how you will laser through your little roadblocks. Create your strategy ahead of time. For example, you might decide to not look at your e-mail and not answer your phone or check messages until you are done with paperwork.

5. Repeat daily and watch how Zoom Focus turns little successes into big results.

44

Have A "Big Bang" Mind-Set

Life is a choice. And every day you can choose to have a "Big Bang" mind-set. You can choose to believe that you create your life every day through your words, thoughts, choices and actions. Where Richard Carlson tells us not to sweat the small stuff, I believe that life is all about the little things. We don't create our lives by focusing on the big things. The big projects, the big promotion, the big car, the big house. Rather we create our life by doing the little things and allowing the big things to happen. If we read one book a week for thirty years, that equals 1,560 books. That's a lot of knowledge. The difference between rain and snow is only a few degrees. They say football is a game of inches. Our lives are no different.

When we have a Big Bang mind-set we accept responsibility for our life. We know that we have the power to create success or succumb to failure. Our life is the result of each choice we make and each action we take. A positive thought leads to a new opportunity in your life. A positive conversation with a group of people leads to a plethora of new friends and contacts. Walking in the morning before work makes

> **"Power is the faculty or capacity to act, the strength and potency to accomplish something. It is the vital energy to make choices and decisions. It also includes the capacity to overcome deeply embedded habits and to cultivate higher, more effective ones."**
> **—STEVEN R. COVEY**

you feel more energized which leads to a promotion. Choosing fruit, nuts, and raisins as snacks instead of candy bars and chips on a daily basis makes a big difference in your health and energy level. Drinking green tea instead of coffee in the afternoon will increase your energy over time and help protect you against cancer.

It's not the big things that you do once that matter. It's the little things that you do every minute of every day that means everything. With a Big Bang mind-set you realize that life is a series of seconds and moments that, when added together, equal your life. You are a work in progress, a creation that is still being created. Therefore, you create your life one thought, one word, one choice, one action at a time.

ACTION STEPS

1. **Focus on your thoughts. Are you choosing positive thoughts or negative thoughts?**
2. **Focus on your words. Are you surrounding yourself with positive words or negative words? Are you speaking positively about life or are you always complaining?**
3. **Focus on your choices. Are you making good choices that benefit you or bad choices that hurt you?**
4. **Focus on your actions. What are you doing to create your life? Do you have a good plan and not follow through or do you take action on your positive thoughts and plans.**

45

Write for Energy

Writing is a great way to create and express positive energy as well as release the clutter in your mind. Try keeping a daily journal. Writing every day is a great way to uncover your fears, desires, thoughts, and dreams—to get in touch with who you are and allow the real you to shine.

Writing helps free up emotional energy and allows new energy to flow in. When you put pen to paper, you release energy from your mind and put this energy on the paper. Writing is a way to project your thoughts to the world. I notice when I am writing I am happier, more fulfilled and easier to be around. Thankfully, my wife feels the same way.

When you write, write for yourself. Don't try to write perfect grammar, or even complete sentences. Just write what comes to mind and release it on paper. Don't monitor your thoughts or make judgments of whether they are good or bad. After you are done writing you can read it. When you are done writing take a few deep breaths and let all the new positive energy flow into your life.

ACTION STEPS

1. Buy a journal at a book or card store. Or use your computer or a pad of paper.

2. Make sure your journal is private, and ask the people you live with to respect your privacy.

3. Stephen King, in his book *On Writing*, recommends we find a comfortable and quiet place to write. Even buy a special writing chair. It's that important.

4. Stephen King also recommends we pick a time each day to write and make it a ritual. Make it a habit. I find I write best in the morning when I feel fresh and rested.

5. Read *The Artist's Way* by Julia Cameron and Mark Bryan.

6. Visit Running Rhino, www.runningrhino.com, to order a journal online or call them at (206) 284-2868.

46

Be Your Own Boss

The most important thing you can do when creating your life is to be your own boss. Everything else feeds off of this one thing. You can't create if you are not in charge of your creation. So repeat after me. I will become my own boss!

Sure, you most likely have a boss at work. We all have to report to someone at sometime in our professional life. Even CEOs report to a group of bosses—their board of directors. However, when you become your own boss you are saying to yourself that you are responsible and in charge of your own energy and your life. Your work boss controls and manages your workflow, work schedule, and other work activities such as travel, meetings, and conferences. On the other hand, you and only you are in charge of your energy, your life flow, your life schedule, and your lifestyle. You may have to be on a plane to catch a meeting in California, but it's up to you to decide how you spend your time and what you eat on the plane. Your boss may give you a certain amount of time to finish the latest project, but it is up to you to incorporate that project into your routine and not let it take over your life.

> **"No bird soars too high if he soars with his own wings."**
> **—WILLIAM BLAKE**

Being your own boss means being an Energy Addict. You are

a conscious, thinking, energized being who is the creator of your life. Any situation, any event, any problem, is taken in, digested, addressed, and mastered. You realize that you and only you are accountable for your life. You stop blaming others for any and every problem in your life and you start making yourself happy and successful.

It's not easy to be your own boss. Many of us would rather have people tell us what to do instead of deciding for ourselves. We might not want the responsibility of being in charge of our own life. It's quite a challenge. It's hard to make the tough decisions and resist temptations. However, once you become your own boss and feel better than you ever have in your life, you will never be able to imagine living any other way. Once you see yourself as both a creator and a creation of your own focused energy, you will seek and grasp the brief moments of time that allow you to create true success.

ACTION STEPS

1. Write down one area of your life where you can take more responsibility for your own actions. For example you might write, "During my lunch break I can make decisions that will benefit me."

2. Next write down several actions you can take that will benefit you during this time. For example you might write, "I will eat a healthier lunch. I will get fresh air during my lunch break. I will take deep breaths and prepare positively for the day ahead."

3. Repeat steps for each area of your life where you would like to be more in control.

47

Master the Flow of Money

Once and for all let's break down money into its most basic form and give it the status it deserves. Money is not a god and should not be worshiped like one. Money, in itself, is not powerful, but it can be used in powerful ways. Money is a form of energy simply waiting to be transformed, exchanged, saved, and used, with its power derived from what it can be turned into. The food we buy, the vacations we take, the lifestyle we live.

Money, like all forms of energy, is used differently by different people. Money can be a friend who helps build a life or it can become an enemy that knocks us down. If you have ever been in or known someone in serious debt, you understand the magnitude of this statement. When used properly, money can provide us with the life we have always wanted—or it can make our world a living nightmare.

Once we simplify how we think about money, we can simplify how we use money in our life. When the public uses more electricity than the power companies produce, we call this a power crisis—an energy deficit. The same can be said for a person who spends more energy than they make. Eventually the deficit grows and a personal crisis results. To master the flow of money, you must master the flow of the energy of money. An energy crisis will not occur if we apply one simple rule to our life.

Spend only what you have. Or don't spend it if you don't have it. I know this sounds overly simplified . . . but face it, we often overlook the obvious. Millions of Americans are in debt because of one thing. They spend more than they make. The law of energy says if you spend energy you don't have, then you will need to find that energy somewhere else. Usually it's in the form of a credit card or loan. Eventually you spend your life trying to replenish the borrowed energy rather than accumulating energy for future needs. If you get to the point where you can't even replenish your borrowed energy, an energy crisis could become a power plant shutdown. The key is to not let the meter go past empty. If input is light, then output needs to be cut back. Whatever the sacrifice, the flow of energy must be balanced and the outflow of money should only increase when inflow increases.

ACTION STEPS

1. **Determine your current monthly inflow (income) and outflow (expenses). Do you spend more than you take in?**

2. **Think of money as energy. If your expenses exceed your income, reduce your expenses so that your inflow is more than your outflow.**

3. **Read *The Wall Street Journal Guide to Understanding Money & Investing* by Kenneth M. Morris. It will help you understand all of the different methods of investing.**

4. **Visit www.fool.com or www.clarkhoward.com for more information on financial matters and ways to save money.**

48

Experience Newness

My eighty-five-year-old grandpa Eddy still writes, plays the piano, and travels the country by train to visit family and friends. To him everything is new once again. He told me once that each morning he gets the local paper and reads the events section. He goes down the list and says, "Yes." "Yes" to a new museum exhibit. "Yes" to a light parade. "Yes" to everything.

I remember a few years ago when I took Grandpa Eddy to the Atlanta Botanical Garden. I watched as he savored the sights and smells of hundreds of flowers and plants with childlike curiosity and awe. I understand now what I felt then—Grandpa Eddy understands that when we are open to new things, new people, new places, and new events we allow more energy into our lives. This energy stimulates our mind and body. It prevents rust from forming and keeps us sharp, alert, fun, and young.

> **"The goal in life is to die young—as late as possible."**
> —ASHLEY MONTAGU, PH.D.

When we lift weights, we notice that our muscles grow in response to this new stimulus. In much the same way, every new experience, every new person we meet, every new event we attend helps us grow into fully energized, fully alive people.

William James said, "We must not just patch and tinker with life. We must keep renewing it." In this spirit let us continually renew our mind, body and spirit by fueling our lives with new experiences.

ACTION STEPS

1. Say "Yes" to everything.
2. Get out of the house and meet one new person this week.
3. Attend the new play or movie that just opened.
4. Go to a museum.
5. Try a new dinner recipe.
6. Take up a new hobby.
7. Buy a new CD.
8. Drive home a different way from work.
9. Learn a new word each day.
10. Take a trip to somewhere near your home that you've never been before.

49

Let Your Energy Shine

In a world of infinite possibilities, choices, and combinations, there has never been, nor will there ever be, anyone like you. You are an original—one of a kind. You may breathe like everyone and talk like most, but your fingerprints are unmatched and your eye's retina is distinct. You are an energy being like everyone and yet everyone is not like you.

Is this scary? I don't think so. I think it's fascinating. What I think is scary is that many of us don't let our uniqueness show. We don't live the lives we were born to live. We don't tap that unique power source inside us. Each one of us is born with a purpose. Each one of us has a unique source of energy to give to the world. It is a gift. When that gift is given to the world we see presents everywhere—Michael Jordan playing basketball, Mozart composing music, Nicole Kidman and Jodie Foster acting, Michelangelo painting, Mia Hamm playing soccer, and Caroline Myss giving a lecture about energy. The list goes on.

> **"Our deepest fear is not that we are inadequate. Our deepest fear is that we are powerful beyond measure. It is our light, not our darkness that frightens us."**
> —MARIANNE WILLIAMSON

But what about the millions of people who don't let their energy shine? Their gifts are still undiscovered in the depths of miserable jobs and unhappy lives. Their light is clouded by the darkness of resentment. Hidden by the desire to fit in and be like everyone else. Masked by settling for a paycheck and the status quo.

How about you? Do you let your energy shine? Or are your gifts still hidden to yourself and the world? Do you know what makes you unique and different? No matter what your gift is, it is important to discover it and believe in it. When you let your energy shine, you unleash an awesome amount of energy that fuels your life and the lives of many others.

ACTION STEPS

1. **Identify what makes you unique and different. Perhaps everyone says that you are one of the friendliest people they have ever met.**
2. **Identify what you are good at. What are you great at? What are your skills?**
3. **Identify what you love to do. What brings you joy? Satisfaction? What jobs do you seem attracted to? Who do you admire and what do they do?**
4. **Spend the time to cultivate these gifts and share them with others. Let your energy shine.**

50

Energize Your Strengths

According to Robert K. Cooper, Ph.D., author of *The Other 90 Percent*, it takes an enormous amount of time, effort, and energy to raise an area of poor performance to mediocre performance. In contrast, it takes very little time and effort to raise an area of good performance to great performance—as long as you're doing something that you enjoy.

Therefore, if we want to maximize our energy and apply it where it will make the biggest impact, we should spend our time doing things we are good at and enjoy. While this seems to be stating the obvious, how many of us spend our time trying to cover up or improve our weaknesses rather than cultivating our strengths? We spend most of our time and energy in the wrong profession or the wrong job doing daily tasks that don't match our skill sets or passion. This mismatch doesn't provide us with an outlet to develop our natural attributes, nor does it allow us to realize our full potential. We waste time trying to become average rather than working to become great. The most successful people identify their strengths and weaknesses, and focus their energies on energizing their strengths rather than wasting their time trying to improve their weaknesses.

> **"Just do what you do best."**
> —RED AUERBACH

When we watch Venus Williams play tennis, Madonna sing, Michael Dell lead a company, or Rudy Guilianni run a city, we clearly see people who have cultivated certain talents that are as natural to them as breathing and eating. The result is that they excel. We can't take our eyes off them. It is no different for you and me. If we know our natural strengths and work to develop these attributes, we too will make the most of our energy and create amazing results.

ACTION STEPS

1. List your skills. What do you do better than most people you know?
2. Write down what you love to do. What activities energize you? Identify what comes natural to you.
3. Write down one of your strengths and list several actions you will take to cultivate this strength.
4. Spend time each day and/or week to cultivate this strength.

51

Be the Age You Want to Be

Baseball great Satchel Paige once asked, "How old would you be if you didn't know how old you are?" Satchel was over 40 the entire time he pitched in the major leagues, but no one really knew how old he was since his birth date always remained a mystery. In 1965, fifty-nine years after Satchel's estimated birth year, he pitched for the last time, throwing three scoreless innings for the Kansas City Athletics. It is said that Satchel rarely answered questions about his age, and when he did he would reply with something like, "Age is a question of mind over matter. If you don't mind, it doesn't matter."

Ask yourself how old you feel. Do you feel younger than your chronological age, but always remind yourself that you are "too old" to be doing this or that? Or do you feel a lot older than you are, and often say something like "I'm getting old. I'm not a kid anymore." I know many sixty- and seventy-year-olds who feel and act younger than people half their age. I also know some forty- and fifty-year-olds who feel and look like they are twenty years older than they are.

No matter what age you are now, you have the option to be the age you want to be. You can feel younger and grow younger at any age. Just forget how old you are and remember how young you want to be. It's all a matter of your mind. If you

> **"Youth has no age."**
> **—PABLO PICASSO**

feel young and think young, you will project youthful energy. When you are open to the possibility that anything is possible at any age, your body will be able to do things you never imagined.

ACTION STEPS

1. **Decide right now the age you want to be.**
2. **Act and feel that you are that age. Observe how your energy increases.**
3. **When people ask you how old you are respond with, "Age is a question of mind over matter. If you don't mind, it doesn't matter."**
4. **Read *Grow Younger, Live Longer* by Deepak Chopra, M.D. and David Simon, M.D.**

52

Forgive

One of the great lessons in life is forgiveness. When we hold on to resentments and negative feelings about people who have hurt, betrayed, or misled us, we literally allow this negative energy to fill us up. This negative energy weighs us down like a ton of bricks and stops positive energy from flowing into our lives.

When I was a young boy, my father and mother divorced. My father remarried and his new family became his number one priority. As is the case with many divorced families, people got hurt—and in this case my brother and I were the ones most affected. As I grew up, the feelings of anger and resentment began to build within me. These negative feelings persisted well into adulthood. I moved away from home and had not seen my father for nine years. We didn't speak. He didn't come to my wedding. Life went on. Then one day after a conversation with my brother, I realized how angry I still was. I realized how this resentment was filling me up. I knew I could never be all that I could be without letting go of this hate.

> **"Holding on to anger is like grasping a hot coal with the intent of throwing it at someone else; you are the one getting burned."**
> **—BUDDHA**

That day, I simply decided to forgive. I called him up; he admitted where he made mistakes, and I understood how tough it must have been being pulled in two different directions. My daughter and I visited him a month later and I felt like a weight had been lifted off my shoulders.

When you forgive, you are not doing it for the person you are forgiving. You are doing if for yourself. When you forgive, you allow more peace, love, joy, and other sources of positive energy into your life. You clear out the bad energy and replace it with the good. You stop being a victim and you start taking control of your own life and happiness.

ACTION STEPS

1. Decide who you need to forgive.

2. Say, "I forgive (the person's name) for doing (what)." Forgive with your words and forgive with your heart. Release your anger and resentment.

3. If the person is alive call them up and tell them that you forgive them. Don't expect a certain response. Remember you are forgiving for you, not for them. If they don't appreciate your forgiveness, don't let this stop you from forgiving. If they're no longer living, write a letter. Remember, forgiveness is for yourself, not for them.

4. Also keep in mind that just because you forgive someone doesn't mean they have to be in your life. While you may forgive someone for their past indiscretion, you are not forced to be their best friend now or in the future.

53

Discover Your "Second Brain"

If you have ever had butterflies before speaking to a group of people, a nervous knot in your stomach, or made a split-second decision without thinking you have experienced the energy of your gut—and this energy is always telling you something if you listen. When I say "gut," I am referring to the enteric nervous system that lives inside our intestines. The gut, or as scientists call it our "second brain," consists of about 100 million neurons, more than our spinal cord. Our second brain is an extremely complex system of nerve cells, neurochemicals that are independent but also interconnected to the brain in our head.

According to the National Institute for Science Education, scientists believe from an evolutionary perspective the brain in our stomach was first to form, because our primitive ancestors were more interested in eating to survive than thinking about what clothes they should wear for the hunting party. When thinking became more important, the brain in the head developed but the brain in the gut still remained. In fact, both brains actually originate from a structure called the *neural crest*, which appears and divides

> **"I feel there are two people inside me—me and my intuition. If I go against her, she'll screw me every time, and if I follow her, we get along quite nicely."**
> **—KIM BASINGER**

during fetal development to and from both of our brains. The complex physical, chemical, and energetic system of the gut enables us to think and act independently of the brain while still influencing the way we think, feel and act.

I share this information with you because the energy of the gut is another power source that can significantly improve the way we interact and excel in the world if we choose to listen to it. Every day our gut sends us messages that can help us in our life. To tap into the energy of the gut we have to be willing to both listen to it and ask it questions. Is this person friend or foe? Should I do this business deal? Is this house a good investment? Is this a dangerous situation? Is this the right time to make the pitch? When making a critical decision, ask your gut what it thinks and listen for the answer. Your second brain actually will have already given you an answer—even before you ask the question.

ACTION STEPS

1. Do a gut check every time you are in a high pressure or tense situation. Communicate with your gut and feel what it is telling you.

2. Practice making decisions with your gut in various situations, under high pressure and normal conditions. The more you practice, the better you will become.

3. For a week, when making decisions write down your gut decision and then write down your rational decision after you had time to think. If they were different, write which one turned out better. If they were the same, write down how you felt about the results. These exercises will help you train yourself to use your gut.

54

Trust Your Gut

Can you think of a time in your life when you didn't listen to your gut and wished you did? We knew our gut was trying to tell us something. Experiencing moments where we have felt its presence but have ignored its power is still an enormous gift—if we look back and know we should have acted with our intuition, then each one of us also knows that we have the ability to tap into the intuitive energy inside us. All we have to do is listen to it and trust it the next time.

When we learn to listen and trust our inner voice, we tap into a source of great wisdom and power. Instead of listening to the fear and doubts often brought about by the rational, thinking mind, our inner voice points us in the direction of our greatest good. This inner voice consists of messages from our gut or second brain and from the energy the great spiritual teachers call our inner knowing or being—that energy inside us that is connected to the infinite energy in the universe or "God" or "higher power." Whatever we call this energy, when we go deep within and connect to this source, our lives will become a miraculous and thrilling ride.

> **"Trusting your intuition means tuning in as deeply as you can to the energy you feel, following that energy moment to moment, trusting that it will lead you where you want to go and bring you everything you desire."**
> **—SHAKTI GAWAIN**

You know the power of your inner voice. Now all you

have to do is trust it and trust often. Be open to the messages and follow them on an exciting journey. I always have fun listening to what my inner voice has to say. And now that I am open to it, and trust it, it has become a part of every decision and success in my life. Practice trusting your gut and observe how you bring more energy and success into your life.

ACTION STEPS

1. Remember a time in your life when your gut told you something and you didn't listen.

2. Think about what stopped you. Usually it is fear or the fact you are trying to please others instead of yourself.

3. The next time you hear your inner voice, listen to it and trust it. Put the fear aside and do what you want to do not what others want you to do.

55

Build More Power Plants

While I don't believe that money can buy you happiness, I do recognize that money is energy—and if you create more money, you create more energy. This energy can be used to improve your health or to improve the lives of others. It can be used to take a trip to the beach or visit relatives in another state. When we don't allow ourselves to become attached to money, we can enjoy having it and spending it. While money can't buy you happiness, happy people can do a lot of great things with money. So build some power plants, make some money, and exchange it for the things that you want. Just remember: Money can't be exchanged for happiness, love, or true success.

> **"Wealth flows from energy and ideas."**
>
> **—WILLIAM FEATHER**

In life, there are those who search for energy and those who create it. My friend Corey decided to be an energy creator. He knew it was time to find other ways to make money besides his weekly paycheck. He bought a condominium with some money he had saved over the last few years, fixed it up, and rented it for more than his monthly mortgage. This one act increased his flow of money by $2,400 a year. After a few years, he had saved enough money to buy another condo. He now had two power plants producing energy. Within a year he bought a third rental property. Then he sold one of his properties and used the profits to buy a more expensive condo that produced more energy. When I last checked Corey had five income producing power plants that added over $25,000 a year to his yearly input.

Keep in mind that I use Corey's example only to demonstrate how one person created their power plants. While real estate came easy to Corey, it may not suit your personality, skill or schedule. The key is to determine what power plants you want to build and then build them. Two years ago I decided to open a restaurant that would support my writing and speaking efforts. I now have three restaurants—or three power plants producing energy. I always lose money in stocks. I am not very good with real estate. But I know how to make money in restaurants. They work for me . . . and you have to decide what works for you. Over the years your power plants will provide you with money for life.

ACTION STEPS

1. **Read *Rich Dad, Poor Dad* by Robert T. Kiyosaki. This book really did change my life.**

2. **Determine what power plants you want to build.**

3. **Save your money and start putting money toward these power plants.**

4. **When you make money from one power plant use this money to build another power plant or a bigger power plant.**

56

Tap into the Energy of Now

Spiritual teacher Eckhart Tolle, author of one of my favorite books, *The Power of Now*, teaches that people are happiest when they live in the "now." He explains that only when we free ourselves from our mind and constant thoughts are we able to experience the power of the present moment. He teaches that our energy is greatest in the now. When we constantly think about the past or the future our energy is both here and there. By thinking of another time and living now, we are essentially splitting our energy and weakening it with each past or future thought. But when we tap into the power of now, we allow all of our energy to be in one place. Not in the future or in the past, but now.

> **"Love the moment and the energy of that moment will spread beyond all boundaries."**
> —CORITA KENT

When we tap into the energy of now we find tremendous power, peace, and happiness. I don't say this as a teacher who is there yet, but as someone who is still learning. I believe we teach what we need to learn and each day I learn to be present and tap into the energy of now. I have found the more often I live in the now, the more energy I have. Living in the past and future can be very draining. With each past and future thought we essentially invest our energy into a vacuum. Energy spent in the past or future is worthless now. It's like investing money in a company that already went bankrupt or hasn't even been created yet.

Ironically, the more we live in the now the more the things we used to desire will find us. Instead of searching, we will be found. This happens because we become a more powerful magnet of energy when we focus all of our energy now. Instead of scattering our energy it grows stronger within us. Other forms of energy such as money, people, and opportunities are attracted to our energy field in much the same manner in which the earth is attracted to the sun.

ACTION STEP

Think of each day as a series of moments. Start by trying to be present in each moment, and practice often. When you are talking to your friend, don't think of what you are going to make for dinner. Only talk to your friend. When you are playing with your kids, watch their expressions. Feel their love. When you do this with increasing frequency a tremendous amount of energy will be created and amazing things will happen in your life.

57

Don't Be a Waiter

I believe everyone should wait tables once in their life so they can learn to appreciate the people who make their living off of the tips and generosity of others. Wait tables once and you will have a new appreciation for the difficulty of this job.

While everyone should try being a waiter of tables, I also believe no one should be a waiter of life. A waiter of life is someone who always waits for everything to happen. Instead of living now and tapping the energy of now, they wait for the future and put their energy into the future. A waiter is always thinking of their next accomplishment, and next vacation. They wait for tomorrow to be happy. They wait for a bigger house, a bigger car, and a bigger paycheck to be satisfied. When tomorrow comes, they are still not content. Then they can't wait to buy a second house and a second car. A waiter so badly wants the future to be now they get very anxious when they are in traffic or in line at the grocery store. Ironically, a waiter of life doesn't wait very well at all. They bang their steering wheel in traffic, make faces at the grocery clerk, and fidget as they wait for an appointment or meeting. A waiter is always thinking of tomorrow so they never enjoy today.

> **"I never think of the future. It comes soon enough."**
> **—ALBERT EINSTEIN**

I still find myself being a waiter at times, but much less than I used to. In the past I was the busiest waiter I knew. I was always thinking of the future. I would project my life into the future and imagine how happy I would be. But I was never happy now. I would often say, "I can't wait until the kids are older. Then we'll have fun." My wife, who is a great teacher, would often respond, "What about now? If you're not happy now, you'll never be happy." Everything changed when I made a conscious decision to give up my job as a waiter of life. I practiced not waiting and like everything in life, if we practice we will get better.

When you give up your job as a waiter you will create more energy in your life. Like we discussed earlier, instead of your energy being split, it will all be here and now. This will allow you to focus on today and now, instead of thinking about tomorrow and the future. This means more energy for our lives and less energy for our future, imagined life. Ironically, when we stop being a waiter the future is better than we could have imagined.

ACTION STEPS

1. Use your time standing in lines to practice not being a waiter.
2. If you often sit in traffic practice enjoying the time in your car.
3. If you find yourself thinking you will be happier in the future, work on being happier now.
4. Read or listen to the book *The Power of Now*.

58

Become a Creator

One thousand, six hundred and sixty-nine hours. That's the amount of time the average American will spend watching television in 2004, according to *USA Today*. That's seventy days a year. Wow.

Just imagine what we could accomplish in seventy days. Unfortunately this statistic brings home the harsh reality that many of us would rather spend hours watching *other people's* reality than cultivate our own optimal reality. Many of us pay our hard-earned money to watch professional athletes enjoy their sport (and become rich doing it), and yet we never engage in the sports ourselves. We help others become rich by buying music, but we never develop the richness of our lives by creating our own music. Many of us watch the Food Network but never cook. We live vicariously through home makeovers, and yet we don't experience the personal joy of sitting down and imagining how we would design our own homes.

The fact is we don't cultivate happiness and energy by watching some Joe become a millionaire or watching some millionaire teach you how to make the best cup of Joe. While obviously there is nothing wrong with watching reality television, cooking shows, sporting events (you'll find me planted in my chair watching Sunday football) and listening to music, the problem lies when we *only* live through other people and fail to create our own reality.

Today I am encouraging you to become a creator. Engage in an activity that brings you joy, excitement and energy. You don't have to cook, play music, write, or throw a football, but it's important to remember to engage yourself with life. I have to remind myself to do this at times. I'll be in my office checking e-mail for what seems like forever, and I'll have to nudge myself and say, "Jon get outside and do something." Just last Saturday I made myself go to the YMCA and play basketball. After not playing for a year I forgot how much I enjoyed it.

What do you enjoy and miss doing? What activity is calling your name?

ACTION STEPS

1. The next time you are watching someone on television showcase their skills, talents, and joy, let this inspire you to discover your own great qualities, skills and happiness.

2. Identify one activity that you want to incorporate into your life. Perhaps it's cooking, writing, singing, dancing, playing golf, inventing, designing, sewing, or gardening.

3. Schedule time each week for this activity. Make time to create.

59

Remember, It's Not a Race

Before I met my wife I was always rushing—rushing to get to the store, rushing to reach my goals, rushing through life hoping to get there faster. While I have learned a lot about life from my wife, the biggest lesson she taught me is the practice of "cruising." Like a car in cruise control, my wife goes at her own steady pace. She eats her meals slowly, savoring each bite. She does the dishes on her own time, not my time. She never rushes to get things done but always manages to get everything done—on her time, at her pace.

While I used to view her way as slow and unproductive (which, you can imagine, led to many arguments), I grew to realize that she knew a secret that I didn't. Instead of letting society and other people, including me, rush her, she dictated her own pace. If the kids would oversleep for school, she wouldn't panic and rush them 90 mph to school as I would have. Instead she would simply bring them thirty minutes late—and believe it or not, life still went on. The sun still set, the school didn't fall down, and the kids still learned their alphabet. I realized rushing really doesn't get things done quicker. While we may move faster or fidget more, we don't make up that much time to call rushing a productivity tool. In fact research states that rushing leads to more mistakes and stress, causing us to work more. Rushing is also a main cause of energy drain.

Just as we use more gas when we try to weave in and out of

cars to get to our destination faster, we also expend more personal energy when we rush. We spend so much energy rushing around we don't have any left when we get there. It's like rushing to a vacation and not being able to enjoy it, or rushing to receive a promotion and not being able to perform because of burnout. In contrast, when you put your life on cruise control you'll find that you'll have more energy every leg of the trip. You'll have more energy to accomplish your short-term tasks and long-term goals. When you cruise instead of rush you still get things done but without the panic and stress.

ACTION STEPS

1 When you find yourself rushing:

- Say to yourself "Life isn't a race."
- Take several deep breaths and relax.
- Pay attention to where you are and what you are doing now rather than thinking about what has to be done and where you have to be.
- Say to yourself, "I have the time to get everything done that I need to get done. Everything always works out when I don't rush."

Make this a habit. If you practice these techniques often they will become part of who you are. You will become a cruiser instead of a rusher.

60

Learn the Energy of "Thank You"

Being thankful has changed my life, and the energy of "thank you" is one of my most powerful sources of energy. Over the last few years I have learned that there is so much to be thankful for and the more we thank the more energy we bring into our lives. When we say "thank you" and feel thankful, we focus the energy of our minds, words, and hearts on what we have . . . rather than what we don't. This energy allows us to be more present, focusing our energy on the *now* rather than the future or negative events of the past.

My friend Jeff told me a story recently about a trip he made to the grocery store. Jeff was tired from a long day's work, and when his wife sent him back out for groceries as soon as he arrived home, Jeff very unwillingly hopped in his car to pick up the needed supplies. On the drive to the store he couldn't stop fuming with angry thoughts and words not fit for this book. Yet, on the way home, he remembered "thank you." He thanked God for the car that took him to the grocery store. He thanked God for the money to buy food. He thanked God for a wife who needed him to buy groceries. By the time he arrived home

> **"If the only prayer you say in your life is 'thank you,' that would suffice."**
>
> **—MEISTER ECKHART**

he was even thankful for the legs to walk and carry six bags of groceries up and down three flights of stairs. When he walked into the door he and his wife embraced, kissed, and life was good. Two simple words changed his outlook on life, his internal energy, and the energy he projected out into the world.

In addition to inner peace, practicing gratitude also attracts more positive people, things, and events into our lives. As in Jeff's case, when you are thankful you vibrate with positive energy and you project this positive energy into the world. Like a magnet, positive people and other forms of energy are attracted to you. It's ironic that by being thankful you actually attract more positive energy in your life than by asking. But that's the way energy works. Each day you have the power to make the energy of "thank you" work for you. Just say "thank you" with your words and feel it with your heart.

ACTION STEPS

1. Say thank you to people whenever you get a chance.
2. Write thank-you notes or thank-you e-mails.
3. Whenever you feel stressed, annoyed or unhappy, remember "thank you."
4. In the morning and before you go to bed, tell God what you are thankful for.
5. Identify three people you would like to thank today and call them or write them.

61

Embrace the Energy of Silence

As I write this I am sitting in my office, looking out the window, and watching a beautiful sunrise. My house is quiet. The kids are asleep and the world is silent, if only for a brief moment. Yet it is in these brief moments that the energy sits, waiting to be tapped, where ideas originate and out of nothing flows everything. The greatest of inventors will tell you that their revolutionary ideas came after moments of silence, just as scientists say that before the big bang all that existed was silence. For all of us, the energy of silence is essential to creating anything meaningful in our lives.

> **"When you're in solitary confinement and you're six feet under without light, sound, or running water, there is no place to go but inside. And when you go inside, you discover that everything that exists in the universe is also within you."**
> **—RUBIN CARTER, THE HURRICANE**

They say it's the spaces between the notes that make the music, and the pauses between sentences that make the speech. Perhaps it can also be said that it's the silence in between the noise of the world that makes our life worth living. Sirens, cars, horns, construction, radios, television, and people all contribute to the constant noise that fills our ears and minds with a bombardment of stimuli. Many days the noise doesn't stop. Yet the energy of silence waits—for that brief moment when the door shuts and the noise stops. Underneath the noise of all things is the silence of everything. Within the silence sits the energy to recharge our batteries—to refuel our tired lives, to help us create.

All we have to do is tap it.

As you read this, you're probably saying, "I don't embrace the energy of silence enough." I urge you now to remember the energy you feel when you close your eyes, clear your breath, and free your mind of noises and thought, and let this feeling inspire you to seek out more silent moments in our noisy world.

ACTION STEPS

1. When you are sitting at your computer, simply stop typing, close your eyes and imagine a beautiful sunset.

2. This one comes from Dr. Wayne Dyer. When driving use red lights as a time to take silent breaks. Close your eyes and free your mind. When the light turns green someone will surely let you know by honking their horn.

3. When you're folding the laundry, enjoy a few minutes of silence.

4. When you are sitting on the couch, turn off the television and embrace a moment of silence.

5. When you walk outside, take a break from your headphones and enjoy a few minutes of walking in silence.

62

Tap the Energy of Thought

Did you ever wonder why so many people seem to have the same idea at once? And how many times have you thought about a friend or relative, and minutes later you receive a call from them? Can all these experiences really be coincidences? They must occur because of the energy of thought. Just because we can't see the energy of thought doesn't mean it doesn't exist. Just because we can't fully explain it doesn't mean it isn't real. We also can't fully explain the way viruses work and we also can't see satellite signals or cell phone transmissions, and yet their energies are being transmitted throughout our world every day.

Thoughts, like all energies, travel and attract other forms of energies like a magnet. The earth attracts the moon. Our cells attract other cells. We are attracted to the energy of other people. Why should the energy of thought be any different? In addition to attracting other ideas, our positive thoughts have the power to attract people, money, jobs, opportunities, good fortune, and many other wonderful things into our lives.

In order to make the energy of your thoughts work for you, you have to stand up and tell yourself and the world what you want. A thought can't travel unless it is born first. To attract what you want, your thoughts must be created, believed, projected and received. To create your thoughts you simply need to think about what you want in your life. What would you like to see happen? What is your dream? Who would you like to meet? How do you want to feel? Where would you like to live? Then you have to turn your wants into beliefs. It is not enough to want things to happen. You have to know that they are going to happen. Thoughts of "wanting" are weak energies. However, thoughts of belief and acceptance are powerful, concrete, and real to you and the world.

The more you believe and accept, the more the world believes and accepts.

ACTION STEPS

Write down five affirmations that are relevant to your life. To help you get started, I have included examples below. As you get comfortable with saying affirmations you will come up with your own style and favorites.

- **I am [your name here]. I accept all the great things in my life.**
- **I am successful. I am happy. I am wealthy. I am healthy.**
- **I accept all the wealth in my life. I accept all the money that flows now through my life.**
- **I accept a call today from ________. I accept the great things we will do together.**
- **Today I will accomplish ________. Today I make it happen. Now is the time. This is the place.**

- I accept all the joy and happiness in my life. I accept all the special people in my life.
- I am healthy. My mind is healthy. My body is healthy.

Focus on these affirmations. Visualize them happening in your mind. Believe that they are a part of your life. Say each affirmation with conviction several times a day.

63

Play to Win

There was a time in most of our lives when we had no fear—we jumped from the jungle gym and slammed our little bodies to the ground, we went on our first roller coaster, and we knew that there was nothing we couldn't do. No goal was unattainable. We were an unstoppable wave of energy; we would think of something and then make it happen.

Then, as time went by, the world told us more frequently that we couldn't do anything we wanted. The Energy Vampires laughed at our goals and tried to dissuade us from going after our dreams. "You're crazy. It's too hard. It's too much of a long shot. Why don't you do this instead? You should play it safe." We not only began to know the word "fear," we started to understand what it was like to be fearful.

Unfortunately this is how many of us go through life. Whether you are twenty or fifty, many of us become so scared of losing what we have that we don't go after what we truly want. We allow the negative energy of fear into our lives, which cuts off the flow of positive energy and paralyzes our desires. We play it safe and hold on so tight to the status quo that we never experience what could be. I call this "playing to lose."

> **"Energy and persistence conquer all things."**
> —BENJAMIN FRANKLIN

To live a life filled with positive energy we must learn to repel the negative energy of fear. Whether it comes from within or from another person we must eliminate fear from our life and replace it with a "play-to-win" mind-set. I have seen this power firsthand. Two years ago, I was working for a technology company, fearful of losing my job and going bankrupt. One day I told my wife, "I'm not going to live like this. No fear anymore. I'm going to do what I was born to do." For me, living in fear was like dying.

Sure enough, two years later, I have three successful restaurants and I am doing what I love—making a difference in other people's lives by sharing energy. I stopped the fear from flowing through my life, and I replaced it with the attitude that I was going to make my dreams come true. Whatever it took, I would make it happen. Once I changed my attitude, positive energy started flowing into and out of my life and everything began falling in place. If I can do it so can you.

ACTION STEPS

1. Identify the fear in your life. What makes you fearful? Remind yourself that this fear serves no purpose. It only weakens you.

2. Use the power of appreciation. According to Dan Baker, Ph.D., coauthor of *What Happy People Know*, research shows that it is physiologically impossible to be in a state of appreciation and a state of fear at the same time. So if you are feeling stressed or fearful, start thinking of things that you can appreciate. Who do you love? Who loves you? Do you have your health? What are you thankful for?

3. Decide to play to win.

64

Live 365 Lives a Year

As I mentioned earlier in the book, my parents divorced when I was a year old. Thankfully my mother married a wonderful person who raised me as his son. My dad was a tough New York City police officer who had hundreds of stories of near misses and close calls. Yet, one particular story has stood out in my mind over the years.

My dad and his partner chased a criminal into an abandoned building. As my dad searched, he moved quietly. The criminal came out of nowhere and placed a gun against my dad's head. My dad's heart began to race, fearing the worst. The criminal then pulled the trigger of the gun. It misfired. My dad's partner was able to knock down the criminal, and they apprehended him. But it changed my dad's life forever. He felt he was given a new lease on life—it wasn't his time to go, and thankfully my mom never had to receive the call she always feared would wake her up in the middle of the night.

> **"I believe I understand life and death. And I am scared of neither."**
> —IVAN GOLDFARB

The truth is we never know when our time is up. The way I see it, if cats have nine lives, then we need to live like we have 365 lives per year for the rest of our lives. In essence, this means that we should begin a new "life" every day. We need to wake up each morning, celebrate that we have been given another life to live, and make the most of that life.

Ask yourself, "If I die tomorrow, would I be happy with the way I lived my life? Would I be proud of my accomplishments? What would my epitaph say? Would I have taken more chances? Did I live my life to the fullest? Did I make a difference in other people's lives? Did I smile enough?"

Your answers will help you focus your life and concentrate on living each day to the max—maximum energy and maximum joy. If you're not satisfied with your answers, the good news is that there is still time to make today count. We can live with boundless energy and enthusiasm for today and only today. We can go for it. We can pursue our dreams and live the life we have always wanted. We can be free to succeed. Failure? Why should we care about failure if we are creating our life every day? At the end of the day failure is dead. Tomorrow begins a new day, a new life, and a new opportunity to succeed.

ACTION STEPS

1. Wake up each morning and say, "Today I begin my new life."
2. Live 365 lives a year for the rest of your life.
3. Ask yourself often, "Am I making the most of today or am I living for tomorrow?"

65

Become a Walking Tourist

This strategy is one of my favorite ways to energize my life. When I go on vacation or visit another city on business I become a walking tourist. Whenever I have the chance I walk around the city and take in all of the energy it has to offer. I see the sights; listen to the noises on the street; hear the conversations outside the corner stores; watch people hustle and bustle about their day.

Once when I was in San Diego I walked about five miles from my hotel to the Coronado Bridge. The sights were breathtaking, and the energy was peaceful. When visiting New York, I have been known to walk ten to fifteen miles in a given day. Instead of taking the time to wave down a taxi, I just keep on walking. On my walks I literally feed off the energy of the city. I look at the different buildings, watch people selling different merchandise on the streets, inhale the aromas from fine restaurants, and delight in the smell of roasted nuts and hot pretzels. I love listening to all of the sounds of the people, places, and machines that create the energy of a thriving city. Before I know it, I have walked for two hours and I'm ready for more.

ACTION STEPS

1. When you're on vacation or business, carve out time in your day to walk around the town or city you are visiting.

2. Instead of exercising in a hotel gym, consider walking around the city or town for your morning or evening exercise.

3. Instead of relying on taxicabs to travel short distances, consider walking a few miles.

66

Become a Walking Tourist in Your Hometown

While it's great to be a walking tourist in a new city, you don't have to limit this exercise to your travels. Sometimes it's more fun to see what's new in your familiar world. I live in a beach community, and I always consider myself a walking tourist. I take long walks and notice that certain houses have added new flowers. One house has been painted; another house is getting a new driveway. Sometimes kids are playing in the street. Many times I'll see the same faces pass me, and some days I'll pass a new face. (Are they visiting, or perhaps new to the area?) I also breathe in the fresh air. I look at the trees and listen to the birds sing and watch the squirrels play. You can actually take the same walk every day and always see something different.

Something new is always happening. We just have to look for it. A walking tourist doesn't walk with their head down staring at their feet. They look at anything and experience everything. A walking tourist with an eye out for something new will never be disappointed. Fuel your life with new sights, sounds, smells, and experiences at home or away from home. For a walking tourist everything is different but the results are the same. More fuel for the mind and more energy for the body.

ACTION STEPS

1. Take frequent walks around your city or town.

2. Look for things that have changed or are changing.

3. Look, listen, and smell while you walk. Engage your senses.

4. Walk with the feeling that you are going to experience something new. When you have this feeling, amazing things will happen.

67

Relax Instead of Talking

The urge comes over us. We are in the car, sitting in traffic, bored as can be. We reach for the mobile phone or turn on the hands-free phone and make a call. Why? Do we really need to talk or are we just trying to fill the time? An Energy Addict knows the difference. The difference between talking unnecessarily and relaxing is the difference between having energy and losing energy. With each meaningless conversation that's only purpose is to fill time, we leak more energy from our lives and prevent ourselves from tapping the powerful energy inside us.

Perhaps we can think of something else to do instead of talk. How about thinking positive thoughts? Reflecting? Relaxing? After all, we're in a car. Isn't that enough technology to handle at once? We should consider using this time to center ourselves; to take deep breaths and relax; to say our thank-yous; to reflect on our professional and personal lives. Instead of talking on the phone to be busy, busy, busy, we can use that time to balance our lives and give ourselves the time and space to energize.

> **"While we may not be able to control all that happens to us, we can control what happens inside us."**
> —BENJAMIN FRANKLIN

ACTION STEPS

1. Try this on your next drive. If you don't really need to talk to anyone, shut your phone off and focus on relaxing while you drive.

2. Take deep breaths while you drive. Focus on your breathing.

3. Thank God for the wonderful things in your life.

4. Observe how you feel when you arrive to your destination. Do you have more energy or less? Notice how you are a safer, less aggressive driver when you do this.

68

Tap the Energy of Information

I know a CEO named Keith Frein, who hired me to give a seminar to his company, PPR Travel. PPR was recently ranked by *Inc.* magazine as the 70th fastest growing company in the United States. After a few discussions with Keith, I realized why his company was so successful—Keith is an Energy Addict who helps his people transform the energy of information into the power of knowledge.

Keith knows in today's world, knowledge is power—and the more you know the more energy you create. So Keith studies, learns, and acquires knowledge. Keith reads books that will help him grow his business. He pays for his company to go to seminars with the thought leaders of the 21st century. He encourages his employees to read books that will help their performance. He reads newspapers, magazines, and online magazines that tell him what is happening in his industry, why it is happening, and what will happen in the future. Keith knows that he must stay one step ahead of his competition and that one step starts with finding the information and using it to grow his business and his life.

Information is like gas in a gas tank. It sits passively, waiting to be used, pure potential energy waiting to be tapped. When we go to the gas pump and fill up we transform potential energy into actual energy for our car. In the same way, when we tap the energy of information we transform it into the power of knowledge. We transform potential energy into actual energy for our life.

In today's world change is not just possible, it is inevitable. You not only need to know about the companies, people, standards and terminology that are dominating the current landscape, but you also need to have an eye on the future. What is coming soon? What could happen five years from now? What could be so disruptive that it changes your entire industry, profession and career or so revolutionary that it changes the way we live? Or what could simply be helpful right now?

The great thing about information is you don't have to be a CEO to find it. In the information age of today, information is cheap and easy to find. Go to your favorite search engine, type a few key words, and you will have thousands of websites and resources at your fingertips. Whether you are searching to improve your career or your life, finding the necessary information is as easy as going to a gas tank and filling up. Just tap the information, learn it, and transform it into the power of knowledge.

ACTION STEPS

1. **Visit www.google.com and use their advanced search feature to find anything you need.**

2. **Read one magazine a month pertaining to your job or career. If you are a full-time parent, study a parenting magazine.**

3. **Subscribe to online newsletters that provide information on topics you want to learn more about. Most are free.**

69

Give Up the Bags

Too many of us carry excess baggage through our life, and this weighs us down like a ton of bricks. This baggage from the past stops us from living energetically, enthusiastically, and joyfully. At times you might say to yourself, *Let it go, it was a long time ago* or *I wish I could just forget about it*, but the past stays with you and holds on to you like an anchor keeps a boat in place.

As we discussed earlier in the book, when your energy is in the past it cannot be in the present. If you put your thoughts and emotions into the past, this means that you have less energy for your life now. Of course you are not going to be as happy, successful, and energetic as you could be—you're only using a small portion of your energy to create a healthy body and healthy mind now. Instead of walking effortlessly, you're carrying around these heavy bags that make you walk slow and tired.

While getting rid of your excess baggage is not always easy, the first step is to be conscious you are carrying around the past with you. Maybe you have a few bags or maybe you have a lot of bags. I have coached people who did not even realize the baggage they carried. Instead of thinking like a winner, they felt like a victim. They thought only

> **"Happiness is good health and a bad memory."**
> **—INGRID BERGMAN**

about who had hurt them in the past instead of who could help them now.

Once you become conscious that you carry too much baggage with you, you can choose to check your baggage—drop it off and let the past do what it wants with it. Consider your life a bus that doesn't allow its passengers to take bags onboard. Bring only yourself, your positive thoughts, your present happiness, and enjoy the ride.

ACTION STEPS

1. Determine if you think too much about your past. Do you identify with your past? Do you think too much about the people and events that hurt you? Do you blame others for your current situation? Do you accept responsibility for your life now?

2. Monitor your words and thoughts. When a past thought or emotion pops up, allow yourself to feel it and think it and then let it go. Don't hold on to it. Forgive the people who have hurt you. Look at the past as a learning experience. Be thankful of what you have now.

3. Don't be a victim. While you have been a victim in the past you don't have to be a victim now. You can take control of your energy and your happiness now.

4. Check your bags at the door and let your past go. Focus your thoughts, words, mind and heart on the present. Decide to create your best life today.

70

Create Your "Yes" List and "No" List

Before we go shopping we create a list. Right? We create lists for everything, from wedding lists to to-do lists. They help us categorize and organize to make good choices. So I thought it would be helpful if we created a positive energy list (yes list) and a negative energy list (no list). This will help you organize your power sources and energy drainers into two easily readable lists.

Life is all about habits. Our words, choices, thoughts and actions are all habits. Thinking positive thoughts is just as much a habit as thinking negative thoughts. So if we want to make positive changes in our lives, we have to change our habits. While replacing a bad habit with a good habit takes time and effort, tools such as this energy list will help you make better choices, remember your priorities and keep you on track.

So let's make a list. On a piece of paper, make two columns. On the left side write at the top of the page "Positive Energy." On the top right side of the page write "Negative Energy." Then simply write down the power sources, under positive energy, that energize your life. Whether you have been incorporating these power sources into your life or whether you want to

> "We are what we repeatedly do. Excellence, then, is not an act, but a habit."
> —ARISTOTLE

make them a new habit, write them down. While you may have a few good habits today, this list will also help you maintain these habits. Under positive energy you might write something like "Eat fruits and vegetables," "Think positive thoughts" and "Drink more water." Under negative energy you might write something like "yelling at family and employees," "gossiping" and "eating fast food."

ACTION STEPS

1. Create your list as long or short as you want it.
2. Write this list on a piece of paper that you carry in your pocket. Also have a copy of this list in your car.
3. Tape this list to your mirror.
4. Wherever you go you will want to see this list to help you make good choices and develop great habits. Remember you are the energy that you fuel your life with.

71

Communicate from the Heart

Would you like to have more meaningful relationships? Would you like to bring more energy into your relationships? I think we all would. In a world getting smaller and faster by the minute, we are finding it more difficult to connect meaningfully with other people. Most of our relationships are based on communicating mind to mind, voice to voice, and head to head, without any heartfelt feeling or emotion into our conversations. We are not giving each other the time or the chance to connect meaningfully.

Real communion and communicating happens when we speak heart to heart. According to Dr. Cooper, researchers have discovered heartbeats are more than mechanical pump pulses; they actually have an intelligent "energy language" that influences how we perceive and relate to the world. Each and every heartbeat is linked to our thinking brain and to the parts of our nervous system that continually influence our perceptions and awareness. Our heart is continually trying to send us messages if we choose to listen.

> "The light that shines in the eyes is the light of the heart."
> —RUMI

When we do listen, we tap into our true power center. According to research published in the *American Journal of Cardiology*, the heart's magnetic field not only permeates every cell in the body but also radiates outward. In fact, electrophysiological changes in feelings transmitted by the heart have been detected up to five feet. This means that if I am standing two to three feet away from you I can feel your heart's energy—your powerful magnetic field—and you can feel mine. That's why we know if someone is being sincere or fake. We can feel it. We can see it. We can read their energy.

ACTION STEPS

1. Engage in meaningful conversations and develop trusting relationships. You'll be amazed at the benefits you receive in the form of advice, life lessons, and positive energy when you spend the time to really talk to people and create real bonds of communication.

2. Practice empathy. Peter Drucker, Ph.D., says, "The number one practical competency for success in life and work is empathy." Empathy means putting yourself in another person's situation: wondering what it would be like to be them, understanding what they are going through, and supporting them.

3. Make eye contact. Rumi said that, "The light that shines in the eyes is the light of the heart." When we make eye contact we expose our heart and communicate more powerfully.

4. Live with passion and enthusiasm. When you live this way you will communicate your heart's energy to others and they will be drawn to your ideas, missions and dreams.

72

Fuel Up with Words

I'm sure you've noticed I have suggested you read several other books throughout this book, and I've listed a few dozen more in the Reading List. I do so because books and words are energy that have the power to inspire, motivate, and energize us. When we fuel up with the right books and the right energy, we function more optimally. We raise our vibration and become more positive. We live more energetically. Read a powerful book and you will never be able to look at life the same way again. Read a book that offers a new perspective and you'll be forever changed. Read a book that motivates you and you'll improve the way you live. Each book you read has the potential to fuel you up with the energy you need when you need it.

> **"One's mind, once stretched by a new idea, never regains its original dimensions."**
> **—OLIVER WENDELL HOLMES**

Visit your local bookstore and see what jumps out at you. I promise, a few books will. I love bookstores and I love books. I believe we really don't necessarily find the books we need, but rather the books we need find us. Every book I have ever read has become a part of me, and my favorite books have changed who I am, what I think, and how I live my life—forever. I urge you to be open to the positive energy of words that will bring a greater source of energy into your life.

ACTION STEPS

1. Go to a bookstore and look around. See what jumps out at you.

2. Buy one book that appeals to you.

3. Make time each day to read it. Even fifteen minutes a day will lead to a lot of books over time.

73

Turn on the Light

We all know what stress can do to us. When our stress rises we can literally feel the energy leak out of our body. Our mind fogs, our heart races and our body slumps. When we are faced with a stressful situation we need to turn on the light.

Just like we turned on the light to neutralize our Energy Vampires, we can turn on the light to conquer our darkest moments. Stress is a negative emotion. It is heavy energy that can weigh us down. Yet it has one weakness. Stress cannot survive in the light. Nor can any negative thought, word, belief, or feeling. The light is too powerful. What is the light? It's that powerful and positive source of love, joy, and happiness that sits inside you.

To turn on the light when you get stressed, try the process below. But remember one thing—to turn on the light you must first *want* to get rid of stress. Many of us say things like, "I'm so busy, I'm just stressed. I have so much to do." What we are really saying is "Look at me. I'm so busy so I'm important and successful." This becomes our story, our drama, and we start identifying with it. It becomes who we are. We have to be willing to give up this mind-set. We have to let go of our story and give up the drama.

> **"I am not bound to win, I am bound to be true. I am not bound to succeed, but I am bound to live up to the light I have."**
> **—ABRAHAM LINCOLN**

Once we do this, we are ready to turn on the light and become energized instead of stressed.

ACTION STEPS

1. Start breathing. Take several energizing breaths. If possible, close your eyes. Stop thinking about everything else and just focus on your breathing. Think, "breathe in, breathe out" to help you focus.

2. Visualize. After a few focused breaths, start visualizing yourself as a calm and happy person while you continue your energizing breaths. Think about what you are thankful for. Think about what's good in your life.

3. Focus on the big picture. Think about your life right now and wonder, in the grand scheme of things, if this problem is really that important. How important would it be if you were sick or dying?

4. Imagine yourself pulling all the energy around you into your mind and body and imagine this energy giving you the strength to accomplish whatever needs to be accomplished. Open your eyes and keep the light turned on. You should feel de-stressed and reenergized.

74

Be an Energy Banker

An Energy Banker makes smart investments with energy. An Energy Banker knows you have to invest upfront in order to see a return on your investment.

Don't sit on the sidelines. Don't be scared of investing your energy in habits, beliefs, and actions that will increase your value tenfold. This is not the stock market, thank God. This is your energy. So be bold and take actions that will help you transform your potential energy into actual energy. Sure, you'll have to expend more energy up front. Taking action requires more energy. But the energy you create as a result will far surpass any upfront investment. It doesn't take a big upfront investment either. A few simple changes and a little extra energy will provide you with big results. The more energy investments you make the higher your energy portfolio will go. Eventually energy investments and big returns will become a normal part of your life and you'll get used to operating at a higher energy level.

ACTION STEPS

1. List all of the people, groups, beliefs, habits and past people and events that receive a piece of your energy.

2. Now assign each investment a percentage out of 100 percent. If you add up all your investments the total should be 100 percent.

3. Then designate each investment as positive, negative, or neutral.

4. Add up your total percentage of positive investments.

5. Then add up your total percentage of negative investments.

6. Identify how much energy you are investing positively and negatively.

75

Tap Your Creative Energy

Where are you when you get your best ideas? This was a question posed by Michael Gelb, author of *How to Think Like Leonardo da Vinci*. Most people say the shower, bed, garden, the walking path or treadmill. Hardly anyone says great ideas come at the office. Robert Frost once joked "The brain is a wonderful organ; it starts working the moment you get up in the morning and doesn't stop until you get to work."

While it may not be that bad, from our own experiences we know that at work we feel more stress, pressure, and frustration. We often try to fight through fatigue, hunger, and deadlines to get the job done. We push harder, work longer, and challenge ourselves every day. But unfortunately the harder we fight the less our energy flows. The harder we think, the less often our great ideas will appear.

Great ideas come to us during a shower because this is when we are usually most relaxed. Think about it. I bet you also have great ideas when you are on vacation. Or when you are driving in your car with the radio off. Or they whisper in your ear and wake you up in the morning. Wherever and whenever your best ideas strike, it is important to understand that it is not by accident. Where stress, anxiety, pushing and fighting block our creative energy, moments of silence, fun, play, and exercise allow us to relax, recharge and connect with our creative force. We are naturally creative beings. We were born to create. And great ideas were meant to pop into our heads.

ACTION STEPS

1. When the pressure mounts and the last thing you want to do is take a break, acknowledge that this is probably the time that you need one the most. Then do it. Do something completely different from the project at hand.

2. Use your energizer breath to focus on your breathing and quiet your mind.

3. Make the time to visit the places where you get your best ideas. Perhaps it's the beach or the mountains.

4. Take a day for yourself and do nothing but relax and read or watch rented movies.

5. Keep a journal.

6. Watch a movie.

76

Believe

I have a white cat named Frankie who thinks he's a dog. He walks around the block with me. He eats dog food. And when I clap my hands and say, "come on boy," he comes running. Amazingly, dogs never chase him. When they first meet Frankie, they always look confused. While the dog looks skittish and nervous, Frankie just sits there calmly looking at the dog, as if to say: "Why are you looking at me? I'm not a cat. I'M A DOG—NOW TURN AROUND AND GO FIND A TREE."

Of course, the dogs *really* know Frankie is a cat . . . but since he is projecting the energy that he's a dog—he really believes it—they don't know what to make of him. After a few encounters with Frankie, the dogs don't seem nervous anymore. Frankie has made them believers and they simply treat him like a dog.

This got me thinking. If Frankie can project the energy of a dog, then we can project the energy of whatever we want to be and how we want to be seen. What if we radiated brilliance and beauty instead of dullness? What if we showcased our strengths instead of our weaknesses? Projected confidence and success instead of insecurities and doubts? Would we feel different? Would others look at us differently? Would they see a dog instead of a cat?

Yes. Yes. Yes. We determine every moment of every day how others view and treat us by how we view and treat ourselves. We are that powerful. The energy we project is the energy we receive. We are like a movie projector and what we project on to the world's movie screen is what the world sees. If you play a success story, your life will be a success. Play a tearjerker and your life will be full of tears. So to receive the energy of everything you want in life, start to project that energy. Know that you are the energy. Believe you are that energy. And that is what you will become.

ACTION STEPS

1. *Create Your Vision*: Create a picture of the life you want.

2. *Embrace Your Vision:* Keep your vision fresh in your mind. Think about it every day. Write your vision down on paper and paste it to your mirror. Don't give up on your vision. No matter what is happening in your life, keep it alive and let the energy brew inside you.

3. *Project Your Vision*: Believe in your vision. Pour your heart into your vision. You have to project your vision using your thoughts, words, and heart.

4. *Take Action*: If you want to be a comedian you have to do what comedians do—be funny. If you want to be fit you have to do what fit people do—exercise.

77

The Gift of Pain

The other day my three-year-old son, thinking he was Superman, decided to jump off a three-foot-high electrical box over our neighbor's shrubs. Ignoring my calls to "get off the box and come here," he caught his foot on the shrub, fell, and broke his arm. At that moment we both learned a lesson in pain. He learned that when you break an arm you experience pain. I learned that when you get angry at someone you love, you experience emotional pain. Both of us learned that pain is truly a gift.

In Gary Zukov's book *Heart of the Soul,* he brilliantly explains that pain is a signal and gift, one that alerts us to the fact that something is wrong so we can do something to fix it. If we didn't have the pain we wouldn't know the arm was broken. In much the same way, anger, frustration, rage, and other negative emotions are a signal that something is wrong with the way we handle difficult situations.

There are only two ways to process energy during difficult situations. Either through trust and love, or through fear and doubt. When my son broke his arm I was angry at myself for not running to stop him. I was upset that he didn't listen to me. I was frustrated that we would have to spend the next five hours in an emer-

> **"I will love the light for it shows me the way, yet I will endure the darkness because it shows me the stars."**
> —OG MANDINO

gency room. Negative emotions were flying through me and out of me. My stomach hurt. My head ached. I was in pain. Using my emotions as a signal (emotions are our body's physical response to our thoughts), I now realize that I wasn't handling the situation very well. I was fearing the worst instead of trusting that everything happens for a reason.

I didn't consider at the time that perhaps this was supposed to happen. Maybe my son's minor injury that day caused him to avoid a more serious accident the next day. Or maybe it happened so he would learn self-control and consequences of his actions. I forgot one of my favorite Richard Bach quotes that says "every problem has a gift for you in its hands."

ACTION STEP

The next time you get angry, depressed, or frustrated, realize that you are being presented with a gift. A signal that something is wrong. Don't ignore or cover the signal like so many of us do. Taking a pill will not fix it. Drinking will only mask it. Being a workaholic will only hide it. Instead you have to pay attention to this pain and use it as a tool to improve your life, improve the way you process energy and deepen your capacity to trust and love. When you learn to trust and love instead of fear and doubt, you will find your emotional pain disappear.

PART 3

SPIRITUAL STRATEGIES

78

Become an Energy Receiver

In my seminars I suggest to people that they go through life with their heads up, their arms out, and their eyes open. I recommend this because as energy beings we not only share our energy with the world, but we also receive a lot of energy from other people and our higher power. When we are open, the energy will find us. It's like tuning in to a great radio station. You adjust the frequency and music will find you.

Unfortunately many of us put up our energy blockers and stop this flow of energy. Many people go through life with their head down and arms closed. They physically and mentally block energy from entering their space. They don't allow life to bring them wonderful unexpected gifts; strangers and friends are not allowed to get too close; and the positive energy of others is not able to penetrate the shield they have built around their life. They don't want or think they need the help of others. They also don't think anyone would want to help them. They fear, distrust, and guard. They build walls to protect themselves, but instead these walls only cut off the supply of energy and lead to a tired and lonely existence. It also takes a lot more energy to keep positive energy out of our lives than it does to let it in.

True success comes when we allow others to share their energy with us. When we open our arms to the world we allow ourselves to receive these wonderful gifts from friends, family, strangers and life. Perhaps these gifts come in the form of a returned lost wallet, a door opened, a check in the mail, g[illegible]t advice, a new perspective on life, a smile, or a new job offer. Or perhaps they come in the form of a sunset, an ocean view, an answered prayer, a family gathering. Each day presents a new opportunity to receive the gifts of life and the gifts of others. When we allow others to share their energy with us and believe that good things will happen, they always will. When we become an Energy Receiver we tune into a more energetic, open and loving life.

ACTION STEPS

1. Determine if and how you block yourself from receiving the positive energy of others. Do you turn away advice? Do you think that you don't need anybody? Are you so afraid of being hurt that you don't accept good friends in your life?

2. Determine if you block yourself from receiving the energy of your higher power. Do you pray for guidance? Do you ask for strength and help?

3. Open your doors and allow new people and new friends to come into your life.

4. Be open to other people's ideas and suggestions without feeling threatened. Learn from everyone you meet.

5. Pray for guidance.

79

Make a Difference

> "If you find it in your heart to care for somebody else, you will have succeeded."
>
> —MAYA ANGELOU

There is a simple law of the universe called Karma that says, "what you give, you will receive" and "if you do good things for others, good things will happen to you." My grandmother used to echo the same belief in one of her favorite phrases: "What comes around goes around."

I believe that it is impossible to truly thrive in life unless we put forth the energy to make a difference in other people's lives. No matter how busy we are and no matter how many things we have going on in life, we need to find the time to make a difference. Not just because good things will happen to us, but also because this is a natural part of the laws of energy and life. Just as we take in energy through food and expend energy through exercise, we also receive energy from others and give energy to the world. We help. We get helped. We give of ourselves to others, and positive things happen to us.

There are many ways we can make a difference. Many people volunteer at homeless shelters during the holidays. We can also volunteer at a women's shelter, at a Boys and Girls Club, or a YMCA. We can become a Big Sister or Big Brother; a member of the Rotary, Lions, or Kiwanis clubs; a coach of a youth athletic team; a guest speaker at a local middle school; a Sunday school teacher at church; or we can fill one of a thousand other roles in our local communities. Many organizations such as The United Way have special weekend volunteer projects especially for busy nine-to-five professionals.

We can also make a difference with our hearts and our wallets. My wife lost both of her parents to cancer, so she is very supportive of cancer research. We can support a local school program. Buy Girl Scout cookies. Give to our spiritual organizations.

We can also make a difference by organizing and planning fund-raisers and creating awareness of specific causes and problems. While living in Atlanta, I started a nonprofit organization called the Phoenix Organization. We united thousands of Atlanta's young professionals to raise money and volunteer for youth focused charities. Through this experience I discovered that it is amazing what we can accomplish when a lot of people give just a little time and a big piece of their heart. The choices are endless and so is the need. When we give we help to fill a void in someone's life, and we fill a void in ours as well.

ACTION STEPS

1. Decide what charities, programs, or schools are meaningful to you. What motivates you to take action?

2. Decide how you would like to get involved. Would you like to fundraise, plan events, volunteer with people, deliver food, etc.?

3. Determine when you are available. After work, during the day, during lunch?

4. Make a commitment to volunteer something of yourself to others.

80

Connect

How many times has it happened to us? We are introduced to a friend of a friend, and that connection leads to a job, a business deal, a date, or even an entirely new life path. Who told you about your job? Who introduced you to the decision maker who bought your product or signed a partnership with your company? How did you meet your significant other?

Many times, our world can get pretty hectic, and the things that help us in life are the very things we stop doing. One of the first few things to go out the window during times of stress is our desire to reach out and meet new people or talk to those we already know. Yet, our relationships and our ability to meet and attract new people into our lives are our most valued treasures and attributes.

Everyone we meet is a potential friend, contact, business partner, or co-worker. When we are open to meeting new people, the possibilities are endless and our world is limitless. The more people we connect with, the more energy we create. Some like to use the "six degrees of separation" concept to describe the idea that we are all connected

> **"The doors we open and close each day decide the lives we live."**
> **—FLORA WHITTEMORE**

Today's world is getting smaller and smaller as communication and transportation becomes cheaper, easier, and faster. Think about all of the almost improbable experiences that happen in your life. You're at the airport, you start talking to the person seated next to you, and it turns out they know your old friend from high school. Or you are in another country and you meet someone who has a cousin that went to college with your brother. You talk to a stranger and find out they know an old friend of yours.

You never know who you are going to meet when you attend an association meeting or professional happy hour. The possibilities are endless when you accept a lunch invitation with a friend, who has someone she wants you to meet. No matter how much work you have on your desk or how many items are still on your to-do list, remember to slow down enough to reach out and connect with new people and old friends. When we connect, we energize ourselves and others.

ACTION STEPS

1. **Call an old friend you haven't spoken to in a while.**
2. **Accept a dinner invitation from your new neighbors—or extend one.**
3. **Host a house party and invite people you want to get to know better.**
4. **Ask a co-worker to join you for lunch.**
5. **If you're a new mother, join a playgroup.**

81

Give the Gift of Energy

Too often we feel like we have to hoard energy, money, the attention of others, the limelight. Greed makes us want more, more, more. We want the biggest piece of the pie instead of making more pies. What we don't realize is that energy wants to be shared. When energy is shared it never decreases. Just as two candle flames held together create a larger flame, two forces of positive energy working together create more energy for everyone. If you have ever been in a brainstorming session or laughed for hours with old friends you haven't seen in a while, you understand the powerful force of energy that is shared and created when we give the gift of energy.

> **"Thousands of candles can be lighted from a single candle, and the life of the candle will not be shortened. Happiness never decreases by being shared."**
> **—BUDDHA**

The key is to think like an Energy Addict and give the gift of energy to everyone you meet, work with, live with, and interact with. Just as energy can be contagious, energy can also be increased and multiplied. Energy Addicts don't hoard energy. They make more energy for everyone around them, and ultimately for themselves. Energy Addicts know that the more energy they give, the more they receive. They don't want a bigger piece of pie; they make the pie bigger. They make their families, organizations, companies, and teams better by giving and sharing their energy. Women like my wife give so much energy to their families they make everyone's life better. People such as CEO Michael Dell, Oprah, NFL quarterback Brent Favre, Steven Spielberg, and author Cheryl Richardson excel in life because they give the gift of energy—and make us all better off.

ACTION STEPS

1. **Treat every interaction as an exchange of energy.**

2. **Identify three ways you can give the gift of your energy each day. For example, "Become a mentor, smile, and encourage others to succeed."**

82

Believe in Miracles

When we choose to believe that everything is a miracle, suddenly our life opens up to a world of possibilities. Our entire state of being changes. Our mood lightens and our energy soars. Like putting on a new pair of glasses, we see the world differently . . . and this view changes the way we think and feel. Instead of a baby we see the birth of a miracle. Instead of a child we see unlimited potential. A simple flower becomes another example of God's amazing creations. Obstacles become hurdles to success. Negative past experiences become learning experiences. Potential energy becomes boundless energy.

> **"There are only two ways to live your life. One is as though nothing is a miracle. The other is as though everything is a miracle."**
> **—ALBERT EINSTEIN**

A belief in miracles is a belief that anything is possible. Any goal is achievable. Wishes are granted and dreams come true. When you believe in miracles you work that much harder with that much more passion and energy because you know it can and will be done. Your belief in miracles awakens your hidden genius and unleashes your awesome potential. You tap your potential energy and transform each miracle into actual energy. While the doubters close themselves off to the energy of all possibilities, your belief in miracles attracts energy to you in order to create the possible. Energy wants to be used—and if you have the will, the energy of what's possible will help you find a way.

A belief in miracles is also a belief that everything happens for a reason. A friend of mine recently said to me, "A coincidence is when God chooses to remain anonymous." I love this quote because I have always believed there are no accidents. Everything is a miracle. Each event, each lesson, each person has been placed in our life for a reason. When we believe in miracles, we see the divinity in everything. All designed to help us become better people. To grow. To learn. God doesn't need to take the credit, because when we believe everything is a miracle, we give credit where credit is due. A chance meeting. A right turn instead of a left. A cancer gone in remission. All are signs that miracles happen every day. If you choose to believe in miracles, they will happen to you and your life will be filled with incredible energy.

ACTION STEPS

1. Read the book *Small Miracles: Extraordinary Coincidences from Everyday Life*, by Yitta Halberstam and Judith Leventhal.
2. Remember any past miracles that have happened in your life. Write them down.
3. Think about the current miracles in your life. Write them down.
4. Ask friends and family to share any miracles that have happened in their lives.

83

Find Signs of Grace

As Chopra says, ordinary people call these clues coincidences. Energy Addicts call them "signs of grace." The funny thing about signs of grace is, at the time, you can't read them. You know they mean *something*, but the sign becomes clearer when you look back at your life with the advantage of some perspective.

Consider the story of the farmer who had a son and a horse. People said, "That's great you have a son and a horse." The farmer said, "Could be good, could be bad." One day the horse ran away and everyone said that was bad. The farmer said, "Could be good or could be bad." Then the horse came back with five more horses. Everyone said this was good. The farmer said, "Could be good, could be bad." While the son was training one of the horses, it threw him and the son broke both his legs. Everyone said this was bad. The farmer said, "Could be good, could be bad." The next day the Army came to take his son away to fight in the Civil War. He couldn't go because both legs were broken.

> **"Seekers are offered clues all the time from the world of the spirit. Ordinary people call these clues coincidences."**
> **—DEEPAK CHOPRA**

The truth is we never know at the time why things happen the way they do. We have two choices. We can look at problems and negative events as problems and negative events, or as learning experiences and signs of grace. When we look at every situation as a sign of grace we live more energetically and calmly. We flow through life and allow our purpose and destiny to unfold. We don't treat every situation as the end of the world. Instead of fighting everything that happens, we accept these experiences and learn from them.

When something unexpected happens in your life, remember: "It could be good, and it could be bad." Instead of getting mad when things don't go as planned, think: "I wonder where this will lead me." And like the farmer's story, when we believe everything happens for a reason our story always has a positive, happy ending.

ACTION STEPS

1. **Think about a time in your life when you thought something bad happened but it turned out to be a blessing.**

2. **Write down each experience and keep this on hand. When uncertainty happens in your life you can refer to these experiences.**

84

Learn Your Life Lessons

> "The trouble I have with you is me."
> —MICHAEL HUSKEY

Do you have events and situations that keep coming up in your life? Do you have recurring themes—issues with control, trust, acceptance, and love—that play over and over again in your life like a broken record? These life lessons will present themselves repeatedly throughout our lives if we don't address them. They will continue to appear in our lives, over and over again, causing unnecessary stress, draining our energy, and creating unhappiness.

For example, throughout the first few years of my marriage I struggled with control issues. I always wanted to control everything. At the time, I saw everything as my wife's fault. She was making me frustrated by letting the repairman charge her too much. It was her fault for not planning dinner. She was to blame for getting into a fender bender. Only when I faced my life lesson—control—did everything begin to change. I realized that the problem wasn't my wife; the problem was me. As new situations arose, I started supporting her rather than blaming her. Not only did she feel more empowered in her life, I felt more empowered in mine. The amazing thing is, once I learned my life lesson, events that "triggered" my control issues actually stopped appearing.

Here's the good news: when we seek to learn from our problems, they simply don't come up anymore. In fact when you see a problem as a *learning experience* instead of a crisis, the problem eventually disappears. When we treat our problems as life lessons and learning experiences, we replace an enormous amount of negative energy with positive energy. Instead of wasting energy on a problem, we create energy by developing a solution. We, in essence, shine a light on our problems . . . and because negative energy can't survive in the light, the problems disappear.

You can identify your life lessons by observing the reoccurring theme in your life. At work do you get into the same arguments with different people? Your life lesson is calling you. Are you drawn into the same destructive dating patterns time and time again? It's time to learn your life lesson. When you do you will spend less energy solving your problems—freeing up your energy for everything else.

ACTION STEPS

1. Identify your life lessons. What issues keep on appearing? Look in the mirror and determine what you need to learn. Be conscious of your life lessons, and seek to change your pattern of behavior when confronted with a life lesson situation. Observe that when you have effectively learned your life lesson they don't come back.

2. Always be on the lookout for other life lessons. You never know when they will appear. Think of every problem as a learning experience and free up your energy.

85

Let It Flow

We live in a changing universe where energy constantly flows from one form to another. The seasons teach us there is a time for everything. In the summer the energy flows to produce bountiful harvests and crops. In autumn, the energy of creation slowly leaves the land as it prepares for winter to recharge. Then winter comes and the land in essence hibernates and reenergizes itself. The land stores up and maximizes its energy to get ready to give life once again in the spring. In the springtime, energy flows and creates vibrancy and liveliness that will lead to a fruitful summer. Each season is essential to the other. And each moment in our life is essential to living the next.

We all will go through cycles in our lives. One month we will feel creative, and the next we'll feel reflective. One day we're happy, and the next we're sad. In my life I have experienced times of surging active energy, and other times I have felt like a bear in hibernation. Yet I realize that each time is as important as the other. We often have to reflect and recharge in order to create. In solitude we can generate energy that can be shared with others during our season of vibrant energy. Sometimes we have to uproot a part of ourselves so that a new life can begin. Sometimes we have to go

> **"There is an appointed time for everything. A time to give birth, and a time to die; A time to plant and a time to uproot what is planted."**
> **—ECCLESIASTES 3:1–2**

through the darkness of winter to experience the lightness of spring. In times of surging energy we need to be active and vibrant, or else the energy will fester inside us. During our times of low energy we need to restore and renew ourselves. We know the seasons will change and so will everything in our life.

The key to maximize your energy is to let the energy flow in and out of your life, from moment to moment and season to season. Don't fight the flow. Fighting the flow of energy is like not allowing the land to go through winter. Without the ability to renew itself, the land will lose all of its energy and lay barren. By not fighting the flow we have more energy when we need it. We must accept how we feel when we feel it. We know everything will come and go, so we must embrace it and let it flow.

ACTION STEP

Think of yourself as a ray of light that everything flows through. Things go through you, and then back through you. You don't hold on to anything. You just enjoy the time.

86

Open Your Chakras

Caroline Myss, Ph.D., in her eye-opening program Energy Anatomy, discusses the Seven Chakras, or energy centers, that exist within our energy system. According to Myss, these Chakras function as central circuits or power centers that run vertically down the center of our body and manage the flow of energy through our energy system.

Whether you believe in the concept of Chakras or not, we can all agree our energetic body, with electricity coursing through our cells and organs, is affected by the flow of energy into and out of our life. When we open up we allow new energy to flow freely through our energetic mind and body without being inhibited by energetic blockages.

> **"Somewhere out beyond right and wrong there is a field, I'll meet you there."**
> **—RUMI**

The way to open up is to simply be open and flexible. It sounds easy, and yet so many people are closed off to new ideas and new experiences that they create their own energy blocks. They don't attempt to meet new people. They don't accept any deviation from "the plan." Living a closed-off life prevents them from experiencing life to the fullest.

To live a life filled with energy it is important to be open and flexible. It is essential to open your mind to new ideas, new perspectives and open your heart to new people. It is vital to expand your mind and be flexible. If an event or situation doesn't go the way you expect, be flexible. If a person doesn't act the way you want them to act, be flexible. It may be one of your life lessons . . . and if you don't learn to be open, your problem will keep occurring. The more you are open, the more energy you will allow into your life.

ACTION STEPS

1. Identify if and how you are rigid, controlling, and closed off.

2. Identify three to five ways that you can be more open. Pick one way to open up and determine how you are going to be more open this week. For example, you may decide to be open to new ideas. This week you will listen to anyone who presents a new idea to you.

87

Tap into the Energy of Love

What would a book about energy be without talking about love? Love, after all, is the most powerful energy source in the universe. It unites and connects. It bonds each one of us to our higher power and to each other. We may feel love when we hold a newborn baby or pet a sweet dog. We may feel it while sitting in church or meditating on the beach. Love is the divine energy that is always present, waiting to flow into your life.

If you have ever been in love, you know the intense surge of energy that pulses through your veins. While we know this kind of romantic love doesn't last forever, it helps us understand the power of love. Although many of us try to tap the energy of love by getting it from others, often in needy and unhealthy ways, the best way to create more love in your life is by becoming a source of love. You don't have to get love from others to feel loved. You can love yourself and know you are loved by God. Amazingly, when you don't search for love, love will find you. By being a lover you will become the loved.

> **"Love never fails."**
> —I CORINTHIANS 13:8

Start by loving the people who are close to you. Give your family love. Then love your friends. They may need love more than you know. If you have a job, love the people you work with. Then love the people who are hard to love. They are often the ones who need it most. It's easier to love a newborn baby or dog, but loving someone who hurts or upsets you demonstrates your true capacity for love.

When we decide to become a source of love, something amazing happens. Rather than trying to search for love, we start to feel it. When we feel it, we share it with others. In return we receive more love from them. This creates more energy for everyone. It all starts with the conscious decision to tap the energy of love.

ACTION STEP

Ask four questions:

- **How can I create more love today?**
- **How can I share more love today?**
- **How can I be open to receiving more love today?**
- **Who needs my love today?**

Answer these questions by your actions.

88

Lead with Your Heart

When I speak to groups, I perform an exercise in which I ask people to point to themselves. Almost everyone in the room inevitably points not at their head or their arm, but right at their heart. That's because the heart is our power center. We are energetic beings with an electromagnetic field within our bodies. Within this electromagnetic field are a heart, a brain, and other organs that run on electrical impulses and energy. According to Dr. Robert Cooper, research shows the body's trillions of cells are strongly influenced by the heart, which generates energy and is in turn, energized by huge electrical fields that engage us with life. In fact, studies show that the heart's electromagnetic field is approximately 5,000 times greater than the field produced by the brain. Our heart is who we are.

> **"The seat of the soul is to be sought in the heart."**
> **—ARISTOTLE**

Unfortunately most of us lead with our head when we should be leading with our heart. The truth is, you can't accomplish anything meaningful in your life without putting your heart into it. Try working at a job without putting your heart into it—you won't last long. Not only will you feel it, but others will be able to see it as well. Try creating something your heart doesn't really want, and it won't happen. A relationship won't last long if you don't put your heart into it. When we lead from the heart, everyone can see it and feel it. Most importantly, so can we.

ACTION STEPS

1. Identify what your heart wants. What does your heart want to do and where does it want you to go? To answer this, ask yourself:

   - What do I love to do?
   - What matters to me?
   - What is my dream?
   - What do I feel passionate about?
   - Who do I love and who loves me?

2. Determine if you put your heart into your work or your life. Do you live with a purpose and do you have enthusiasm for what you do? If you don't have a sense of purpose now, can you find it in your current work? When my wife refers to her job as the caretaker of our children, she says she is not just raising her children. She is raising them to be future leaders and healers. To me, her job is filled with the ultimate purpose.

3. If you can't find a sense of purpose in your current work, consider finding a job or career that gives you a sense of purpose. Seek out people you admire and find out what they do. What jobs are you naturally attracted to? Start here.

89

Tap Your Share of Infinity

No one really knows how big the universe is. But no matter what the scientists approximate, we can all agree that the universe is big. Really big. And if we know the universe is big we must also assume that there is a whole lot of energy in the universe—and there is.

The way I see it, God is a BIG GOD with a lot of energy. Perhaps an infinite amount of energy. This energy makes the world go around. It lights up the stars and fuels every living creature on earth. With so much energy in the universe, and with such a big God, I often wonder why many of us expect so little of ourselves and the world around us.

As an Energy Addict we must tap our share of infinity. There is so much energy in the universe—even if we tap a big share, there will still be plenty of energy for everyone else. Don't be afraid to ask for more energy than you think you deserve. You deserve everything you need. You are a shining star, and you need lots of energy to shine your light. This doesn't mean that you are greedy. It means that whatever you want to create in your life, you can expect to have the energy to make it happen. You are not afraid to ask God for what you need to do great things in this world. You realize when you expect more,

> "You are never given a wish without also being given the power to make it true."
> —RICHARD BACH

you get more and you do more. God wants you to have it and wants you to use it.

Make this moment the last time you think a dream will not happen. Understand this energy comes in many ways and takes many forms. Believe God and the universe will provide you with all the energy you will ever need to accomplish your goals and live your dreams.

ACTION STEPS

1. Decide what you want to do or create. What is your goal?

2. Expect God will provide you with the resources you need. Don't even doubt it for a second. Believe that it is happening right now.

3. Take action. Put all of your energy in the present moment to reach your goal. Set the wheels in motion. Put your energy out there. Watch how the pipeline opens and you receive your share of infinity.

90

Love Life

It was a profound moment. His name was George and he was a bus driver. George was taking me and a few other men to the Denver airport from the rental car lot, and he had a smile on his face the entire time. He told us jokes. He laughed at ours. When I got off the bus I had to ask him the question—"George, why are you so happy?"

He didn't hesitate. He didn't waiver. Eye's shining, smile beaming, George said in a booming voice, "Because I LOVE LIFE." Then he said it again. "I love life. I love you, I love God, I love myself." Then he added, "How can I love myself if I don't love you? How can I love myself if I don't love God? Everything's connected. I love it all." With that he said have a great trip and I went on my way, forever changed with George's words in my heart. We certainly are all teachers and students.

So how can we love life? What does it mean to love life? While we can't measure the infinite, indivisible, unquantifiable force of love, we certainly can tell when it is present. I think of my grandmother who loved her family so much you could literally taste the love she poured into her meals. I think about CEOs I have met who love their companies and people so much you can notice the difference immediately. I think about moms I have coached who love their children so much you can see it in their kid's eyes. I think about people who seem to flow through life effortlessly because they are in joy. So I believe to LOVE LIFE is to bring love into the present moment—no matter where you are and what you are doing. Whether you are driving a bus, cooking, or working at a desk, to LOVE LIFE is to LOVE the very essence of being alive. To experience joy that you are living. To love everybody and all things. To know that at any moment it can all be taken away, and to appreciate every day, every minute, every second, and every moment of life.

ACTION STEP

Gather five–ten blank sheets of paper. In large letters write on each sheet of paper, "I LOVE LIFE." Now place these signs in places that you will see them throughout the day—your bathroom mirror, your car dashboard, your desk, your office break room, your refrigerator. As you go about your day these signs will help serve as a reminder to LOVE LIFE.

91

Challenge Life

As I talked with my eighty-five-year-old grandpa Eddy the other night, he told me that he still likes mowing his lawn. "I mow the front first. Then I take a break and mow the back. I look at it as a challenge not a chore," he said. "When mowing my lawn becomes a chore and I have trouble doing it, then I'll ask for help."

How many of us go through life as if it's a chore? We drag ourselves out of bed, into our cars and to our jobs. We struggle through life either resisting the power and potential of the present moment or passively accepting our current situation—like a child being told by his father to weed the lawn. Yet what if we took on life as a challenge instead of a chore? I believe we would see life as a series of choices, obstacles, hurdles, and successes. We would challenge life, instead of life challenging us. Like an olympic hurdler, we would grow stronger and more powerful with each hurdle behind us. We would flow through life with a smile instead of a frown.

But what about when life IS a chore? Eddy knows at some point mowing his lawn will become a chore—maybe when he hits 95 or 105! And we must realize life will at times become a chore despite our best intentions and positive energy. So how can we make the transition from "chore" to "challenge" when facing the most difficult times in our lives? Like Eddy, we must ask for help.

ACTION STEPS

1. First ask God for help. When you ask God for help you open the pipeline to an infinite supply of spiritual energy and support. To ask for help simply say "I pray for guidance. I pray for the strength and support to get through this." You'll be amazed at the results.

2. Next ask your friends and family for help. We need other people, and their support and energy can help carry us over the mountain and allow us to run down the hill.

3. And finally ask yourself for help. Appeal to your inner power. Wake up the part of you that wants to shine. It's there, no matter how low you might feel. Encourage yourself through self-talk. Say, "I have the strength to get through this. I know I can do it." Instead of sabotaging your life with negative self-talk become your own positive energy coach and help yourself overcome any obstacle.

92

Remember Your Big Life Plan

It's big but you can't see it. So great that if you could see it you wouldn't believe it. It's your destiny and it's calling you. I call this your Big Life Plan.

Every day we face challenges, fears, obstacles, and negativity that hit us with left jabs and right hooks. We get so caught up in the details of bills, job pressures, raising kids, fixing the house, car payments, trying to make a living and a hundred other to-dos, that we can't even see over the piles of paper on our desk—never mind our future success. But when times are tough and your bills are bigger than the balance in your checking account, remember that there is greatness in you. There is a Big Life Plan for you.

Your destiny sits inside your soul like DNA sits inside your genes. You may not be able to see it, but it's there—waiting to unfold if you let it. Don't let yourself get caught up in the crashing waves. Instead jump those waves and keep your head up, looking out into the horizon. And if you experience a wave so big that there is no way you can jump it, then ride it. Learn from the surfer who challenges wave after wave, growing stronger, developing more balance, and becoming more skilled every day. A smooth ocean never made a skilled surfer and a struggle-free existence never made a meaningful, great life.

ACTION STEP

The next time you are facing a difficult situation remember that there is more than what is in front of you. There is a challenge, a lesson, and a plan. Emerson said "The wise man in the storm prays to God, not for safety from danger, but for deliverance from fear." Don't let fear get in the way of the life that is meant for you. Trust that there is a plan for you and let the possibilities unfold. In the process you will discover the great things you are born to do. You don't have to push. Just trust and your destiny will meet you when the time is right.

93

Build a Bridge . . .

Whether we're planning to make a long-awaited change in our lives or just starting in the pursuit of a dream, the gap between where we are and where we want to be often seems insurmountable. It's like standing at the edge of a cliff and seeing the wonders that await you on the other side. Yet the rational and fearful part of your mind says, "Don't do it. The chasm is too great, too wide. You'll never make it. You'll fail."

In life we face many gaps, and too often we let fear and paralysis stop us from jumping to where we want to be. We resist and stay where it's safe and predictable. We often let the dreams we had when we were young fade into the prisons of responsibilities, paychecks, and mortgage payments. We watch others make the jump and think, *That could be me* . . . but we walk away from the cliff, hands folded, thinking, *Maybe tomorrow will be the day*. We know something has to change. We can feel the energy becoming stagnant. We're ready, but how do we get through the wall of fear?

In times such as these, two components are needed—a bridge and a leap of faith. Since it doesn't make sense to just jump without thinking or planning, building a bridge helps you connect the side of where you are to the side of where you want to be. A bridge helps you get a little closer to the other side and gives you a better view of where you'll land when you make your jump.

ACTION STEPS

1 *Research and gather information*. This helps you transform any risk into a calculated risk. Ask and answer questions depending on your situation. What will it take to receive a promotion? How much does it cost to start my own business? Who is my competition? What are the benefits if everything goes right? What's the worst-case scenario?

2 *Take a survey*. Ask a bunch of people you respect what they think. Learn from what they say, but don't let their opinions sway you completely. When I first decided to open a restaurant, run for city council, and start a nonprofit organization I had many people tell me I was making a mistake. On each occasion some said go for it, while others said no. With each person I considered the source and the advice.

3 *Gut check*. Ask your gut what it thinks. Your first instinct, before you have time to think about it, is often your best decision maker. We talked about this concept earlier. Too often we override our gut instinct because of fear.

4 *Heart check*. It is impossible to accomplish anything meaningful if your heart is not behind it. If your heart is not into it, don't do it.

Finally, after you weigh all the information, it's time to decide whether to take a Leap of Faith.

94

. . . And Take a Leap of Faith

Once you decide to jump and you've built as strong of a bridge as you can, then it's time to take a leap of faith.

When you jump, believe without a doubt that you will land on the other side. Sure you'll scrape a leg here or there. But have faith. Have no fear. (It's not called a leap of fear!) It's called a leap of faith.

Believe that you will attract everything you need to make your leap successful. The energy we project is the energy we receive. Don't listen to the Energy Vampires. They'll try to discourage you during the middle of your jump. They'll try to make you think you won't make it unless you follow their rules. Rules that say things like: your resume has to be a certain way to get hired. Or you have to take a cooking class to become a cook or a writing class to become a writer. But we don't have to be guided by their set of rules. Who makes these rules anyway? They never worked for me.

During our leap of faith we need to follow a different set of rules—guidelines that, instead of confining our growth, allow us to flourish. These rules say: When it is time for you to make it happen, you will. You may not know how to do everything but you can learn. The future is unpredictable but if you are flexible, alert, persistent, and you believe in your heart that this is your path, then everything will work out. Visualize success and you will create it. Be open to receiving guidance and you will receive it. You'll be amazed with how many people come out of the blue to help you.

Let go and let it flow. Have faith and realize you're not in control. Believe you were meant to take this leap of faith and you deserve all the wonderful things that come from it. Remember, it's not the leap that matters the most. Each one of us will take different kinds of leaps throughout our life. The key is how we approach the leap. So fuel your tank with ambition, positive energy, goals, and dreams. Build that bridge, take your leap of faith, and I'll see you on the other side.

ACTION STEP

Armed with knowledge you gained from the "bridge" you just created, take a leap of faith.

95

Choose Love

As I walked off the airplane yesterday and watched a daughter hug her mom, a man get tackled by his wife and kids, and two sisters hug as if they hadn't seen each other in years I was struck by a simple, powerful fact. Despite all the evil, turmoil, and hatred in the world, LOVE IS ALL AROUND US.

Anyone who has witnessed the birth of a baby knows that we come into this world with love. And if you have ever been at the bedside of a dearly departed loved one, you know we leave with love as well. The real question, however, is: Do we love during the time in between? Do we feel love? Do we give love?

We must look inside and ask if we are feeling, expressing and sharing the love inside us. Ultimately we decide to love or not to love. We can choose to see the love that is all around us or choose to ignore it. We can choose to express the love we are born with or choose to hide it.

ACTION STEPS

1. *Love yourself*. Practice self-care. You deserve it. Get a massage. Make yourself a special meal that a loving mother would make you. Buy something that you have always wanted and recognize this act as a gift of self-love. Pick a day and do something fun and special for yourself. Stop beating yourself up. Love all of yourself—even your imperfections.

2 *Become a love magnet*. You don't do this by wearing cologne or perfume. Rather it happens when you become a source of love. We often think that we need to go out of our way to make people like us and love us, but in reality all we have to do is simply love others. When you love others and share love, ironically you will receive all the love you have ever wanted. When you project "needy" energy based on a desire to be loved, the harder you will have to work to be loved. Yet, when you become a lover who loves for the sake of truly loving others, rather trying to receive it, love will flow into your life.

3 *Choose love*. When someone gossips about a friend—choose love. Gossip is wasted negative energy anyway. When someone yells at you—choose love. When someone talks of hate—choose love. When someone wastes his or her energy on anger—invest your energy in love. When you get down to it, it really is a simple choice. When you choose love you bring more happiness, special people, opportunities, and positive energy into your life.

96

Pray for Guidance

In the book *The Greatest Salesman in the World*, Og Mandino writes we should pray for guidance. This simple lesson changed my life more than any lesson I have ever learned.

A few years ago, I was working for a technology company. But I had a feeling the company might be heading toward difficult times—nothing definite, just something in the air—so I started considering other options. Having been in the restaurant business in the past, I decided to get back into it with the hopes it would do well enough to give me the time to write, teach, speak and coach. I did my homework, lined up financing, and laid all the groundwork for my restaurant to open while I was working for the technology company. A week before the restaurant was scheduled to open, I received the call. My boss was on the other line. My hunch was right—I was about to be "downsized."

At first I went into panic mode. What about my family? Insurance? Bills? Then I thought about the restaurant. Thank God I had put a plan in place. But what if the restaurant failed? What if it didn't make money? What would I do then? With all these thoughts running through my mind, I felt powerless. For a control freak like me, this was not a pleasant feeling. But at that very moment I knew I had to let go. I surrendered. I

> **"Take the first step in faith. You don't have to see the whole staircase, just take the first step."**
> **—DR. MARTIN LUTHER KING JR.**

prayed for guidance. I had no choice. Everything was in God's hands.

I chose to believe I was fired at this moment for a reason, and I would be provided for if I had faith. In fact, I soon realized there was a great reason for me being fired. Instead of thinking about a day job, I was able to pour my full energy into making the restaurant successful. We broke even the first week we were open. I then opened two more restaurants and built a management team to run them so I could do my life's work—writing, speaking, and coaching people on energy. I continued to pray for guidance. I started an online newsletter offering energy tips. Soon the list grew and grew as people e-mailed each other. One of my e-mails made it to a publisher. He thought people needed to hear what I had to say, and so he decided to publish this book.

And now, I am here today helping people energize their lives, making a difference, and doing what I love to do. I realize the day I was fired, I was being guided. When I let go and put my trust in God I allowed my purpose and my life to unfold. I hope my story will help you realize when you pray for guidance you tap into your highest and higher power and greatest source of wisdom and energy. No matter what your religion may be, there is one universal source of energy that will guide you where you need to go if you ask, if you let go, if you surrender, and if you let yourself be guided. The fact you are reading these words right now tells me you will soon experience this for yourself.

ACTION STEP

Pray for guidance. You might say, "God, please guide me on my life's path. I pray that you will guide me and help me live my purpose. Give me the strength to get through this difficult time and show me the way to my higher purpose."

CONCLUSION

SHARE THE ENERGY

97

Plant New Energy Seeds

As a child I watched my dad plant tomato seeds every spring in our little backyard garden. And as spring turned into summer I couldn't help but notice these seeds turning into bountiful tomato plants.

Years later I am reminded of a different kind of seed that yields a different kind of harvest. I call these seeds positive energy seeds and they come in the form of positive thoughts, words, and actions. With every thought, every word, and every action, you are planting your energy seeds into your home, office, world and universe. Like a tomato seed your positive energy seeds will grow into something that nurtures and thrives. Calling a friend who is struggling will brighten their day. Engaging in a random act of kindness will make a difference in someone's life. Even simply thinking positive thoughts at home will energize your family.

However, with energy seeds (unlike with a tomato seed) you may not always get to see the fruits of your labor. While you may cultivate positive energy seeds, you may not see the impact it has for months, years, or in many cases, ever. At times this can be frustrating—we like instant gratification! We're human. We want to know that our actions are creating immediate results. Yet, when it comes to energy seeds, the harvest may

> **"With every deed you are sowing a seed, though the harvest you may not see."**
> **—ELLA WHEELER WILCOX**

take place somewhere else, far away and far into the future. Your child may thank you twenty years later for something he or she didn't appreciate at the time. A stranger you help today may save someone's life ten years from now. Your generosity toward someone in need may impact that person's children and their children and future generations to come. Have faith that you are making a difference, even if you never see the harvest. We must plant our seeds not for the desire to see results, but with the faith and knowledge that they will produce a harvest somewhere, sometime, and make a difference somehow.

ACTION STEPS

1. *Plant energy seeds.* Spend your time and energy thinking positive thoughts, being kind, making a difference and helping others. Don't worry about immediate results. Just be an energy seed planter and plant, plant, plant. Visit www.giftofkindness.com for ways to make a difference.

2. *Send seeds of love.* Send a card, e-mail, or make a call to at least five people this week. Simply say, "I was thinking about you and just wanted to send my love."

3. *Project compassion.* Try this today. As you walk down the street or through your office or around the grocery store, as you notice people sitting, standing or walking, silently wish them well. I tried this

as I walked down Fifth Avenue in New York City last week as hun-
did I feel like I was making the world more positive (just imagine if millions of people did this each day) but I am also activating the part of my brain associated with positive emotions—making me happier and more energetic.

98

Surround Yourself with Other Energy Addicts

My dad used to say that you can tell a lot about a person by who they surround themselves with. He was more right than he could have known. The people we surround ourselves with have the potential to give us a boost of energy or zap our energy. If you have ever had someone encourage you to "go for it" and "make it happen" or given you ideas and positive feedback, you know how we can be energized by others. On the other hand, if you have had someone tell you to "give up" and "you don't have what it takes" or made you feel inferior, you know how this can potentially fill us up with negative energy and doubts.

> **"When I find myself fading, I close my eyes and realize my friends are my energy."**
> **—ANONYMOUS**

Who do you surround yourself with? Do they fuel you up or drain the life right out of you? As we discussed earlier, an important key to becoming an Energy Addict is ridding your life of Energy Vampires and finding other Energy Addicts to support you.

No one lives in a vacuum. We need each other. It takes more than one instrument to make a symphony, and it takes more than nine players to make a baseball team. And even golf and tennis players need guidance and support from coaches. Who you surround yourself with says a lot about you and how much energy you want to have. Instead of wasting time and energy trying to convince the people who don't believe in us, we need to spend more time with the people who support us. The key is to identify these people and make time to spend with them.

ACTION STEPS

1. Determine who helps you increase your energy. Who is a positive source of energy in your life?

2. Find ways to spend more time with these people. For example, make a date night each week to go out with your significant other, make Saturday night friends night out, or meet a mentor for lunch or breakfast every Monday.

3. Identify five ways to energize a friend, family member, co-worker, or employee. Start now and ask them to do the same.

99

Start an Energy Addict's Club

Consider all the 12-step groups and organizations that support people in their struggles with bad relationships, substance abuse, addictions, deaths, and diseases. While these groups and organizations serve a wonderful purpose in society, why should we only rally around each other in times of trouble? What a great idea it would be to create a support group to help each other fuel our lives with positive energy and positive habits.

Imagine a group of people getting together once a week or once a month and discussing ways to improve each other's lives. Imagine sharing positive energy and success stories, as each person learns new strategies and tips. Envision the difference you will make to the people who are just getting started. As an Energy Addict, you can help others find more energy in their own lives.

The legacy you can leave doing this is enormous. Imagine the energy this group will create in your town or city. Envision the power of a group of positive people who are addicted to positive energy. What benefit will this have on the community? And imagine this group increasing the physical, mental, and spiritual energy of

> **"Never doubt that a small group of thoughtful, committed citizens can change the world. Indeed, it's the only thing that ever has."**
> **—MARGARET MEAD**

each of its members, its members' families, friends, and co-workers. Think about people like you and me starting this club at work or in our community.

OK, enough convincing. Let's get started. If you are interested in starting an Energy Addict's Club, take the following steps.

ACTION STEPS

1. Gather a few interested people together. Consider holding monthly meetings and keeping in touch between meetings with weekly phone calls. Possible venues: someone's house, a church, school, banquet room in a restaurant.

2. At each meeting, ask each member to stand up, say their name, and say "I am an Energy Addict. I have been an Energy Addict for ________ amount of time." Visitors can introduce themselves and say why they are there.

3. The meeting can vary each week. Perhaps someone shares a personal growth story. A speaker can attend and share new insights. And during each meeting, the group discusses one or more tips to increase your physical, mental, and spiritual energy. Members share how they have incorporated this tip or how they plan to incorporate this tip into their life. They might discuss obstacles that came up and how they overcame them. Tips are taken from this book or new tips are developed and offered by the members.

4. E-mail me at jon@jongordon.com or call 904-285-6842 and we will guide you through the process. It's very easy and of course there is no charge. Together we will spread positive energy.

100

Sponsor Someone

A significant component of any addiction group is the concept of a sponsor. A sponsor is there to support someone through the process of their recovery. The sponsor has been through the program and can offer personal experiences that guide and support the person as they face various obstacles. As an Energy Addict you can offer a great deal of wisdom, insight and experience to others as they then become addicted to positive energy. Your energy is contagious and by working with others as a sponsor you can help them increase their energy. You can help them focus to create what matters most. And you can help them discover simple, powerful ways they can energize their life.

The key is to sponsor only the people who want to be sponsored. Just like AA, you can only help people who want to help themselves. Simply ask someone if they would like to have more energy in their life. Most people will say "yes." The next step is to tell them they should read this book. Give them a copy of your book, tell them to go to the library and check it out, or even buy one for them if you can afford it!

> **"If you can't feed a hundred people, then feed just one."**
> —MOTHER TERESA

ACTION STEP

Find someone who wants your support and help during their process of becoming an Energy Addict. Tell them they can ask your advice anytime. And when you give advice, do so with compassion. It's important to let the person know that you have been through this process and you understand the significant changes they are making in their life. As the person becomes an Energy Addict you are there to support, guide and advise them. They will feel your energy and support and will likely reach new heights because of you.

In turn this person will be equipped to sponsor someone else. Eventually we will have Energy Addicts around the country living and helping others live a life filled with positive energy and positive habits. It all starts with becoming an Energy Addict ourselves. Then we can make a difference by sponsoring someone else.

101

Be Contagious

Positive Energy Addiction is one addiction we want to be contagious. In sports, winning is contagious. Losing is contagious. And positive energy is contagious.

Because we are connected to so many people, each day we have the opportunity to be contagious and share positive energy with those near to us and those far away. A pat on the back to a co-worker can make all the difference. A compliment to a friend can change their entire day. A smile and a kind word to a grocery clerk can have ripple effects beyond your imagination. Who knows how many people the grocery clerk made laugh and smile because of you? And who knows how many of those people went home and were nicer to their children? When I e-mail my newsletter to thousands of people I often wonder who it has been forwarded to and how it has impacted their lives. I don't even know them and yet my positive energy has been shared with them. In writing this book I hope to share positive energy with you in the hope you will share it with others. Together we can be contagious and spread positive energy to our co-workers, family, friends and strangers. And so on and so on.

> **"The world is like a mirror, you see? Smile and your friends smile back."**
>
> **—JAPANESE ZEN SAYING**

ACTION STEPS

1. Be contagious.
2. Remember to smile and smile often.
3. Give hugs (when appropriate), pats on the back, handshakes and high fives.
4. Compliment people often.
5. Make others feel good about themselves while being sincere.
6. Share good news, great stores and happy endings with your co-workers and/or family.

READING LIST

Baker, Dan and Cameron Stauth. *What Happy People Know*. Emmaus, PA: Rodale, 2003.

Cailliet, Rene and Leonard Gross. *The Rejuvenation Strategy*. New York: Doubleday, 1987.

Chopra, Deepak. *Perfect Health*. New York: Three Rivers Press, 2001.

Chopra, Deepak and David Simon. *Grow Younger, Live Longer*. New York: Three Rivers Press, 2001.

Cooper, Robert. *High Energy Living*. New York: New American Library, 2002.

Dyer, Wayne. *10 Secrets for Success and Inner Peace*. Carlsbad: Hay House, 2001.

Grandjean, Etienne. *Fitting the Task to the Man: A Textbook of Occupational Ergonomics*. London: Taylor & Francis, 1988.

Mark, Vernon and Jeffrey Mark. *Brain Power: A Neurosurgeon's Complete Program to Maintain and Enhance Brain Fitness Throughout Your Life*. Boston: Houghton Mifflin, 1989.

Moore-Ede, Martin. *The Twenty-Four Hour Society*. Reading, Mass: Addison-Wesley, 1993.

Myss, Caroline. *Sacred Contracts*. New York: Harmony Books, 2001.

Rossi, Ernest Lawrence. *The 20-Minute Break*. Los Angeles: Tarcher, 1991.

Scott, Susan. *Fierce Conversations: Achieving Success at Work & in Life, One Conversation at a Time*. New York: Viking Press, 2002.

Thayer, Robert. *The Origin of Everyday Moods: Managing Energy, Tension and Stress*. New York: Oxford University Press, 1997.

Tolle, Eckhart. *The Power of Now*. Novato, CA: New World Library, 1999.

Weil, Andrew. *Eating Well for Optimum Health*. New York: Quill, 2001.

Williamson, Marianne. *Everyday Grace*. New York: Riverhead Books, 2002.

CONTACT THE ENERGY ADDICT

I would like to thank you for allowing me to share my energy with you. I hope it makes a difference in your life. I wish you all the best and may your life be filled with boundless energy. Please e-mail me and let me know how you are doing: jon@jongordon.com.

Check out the Energy Addict lifestyle on the Web at www.energyaddict.com.